NO PAIN NO GAIN!

Training Journal

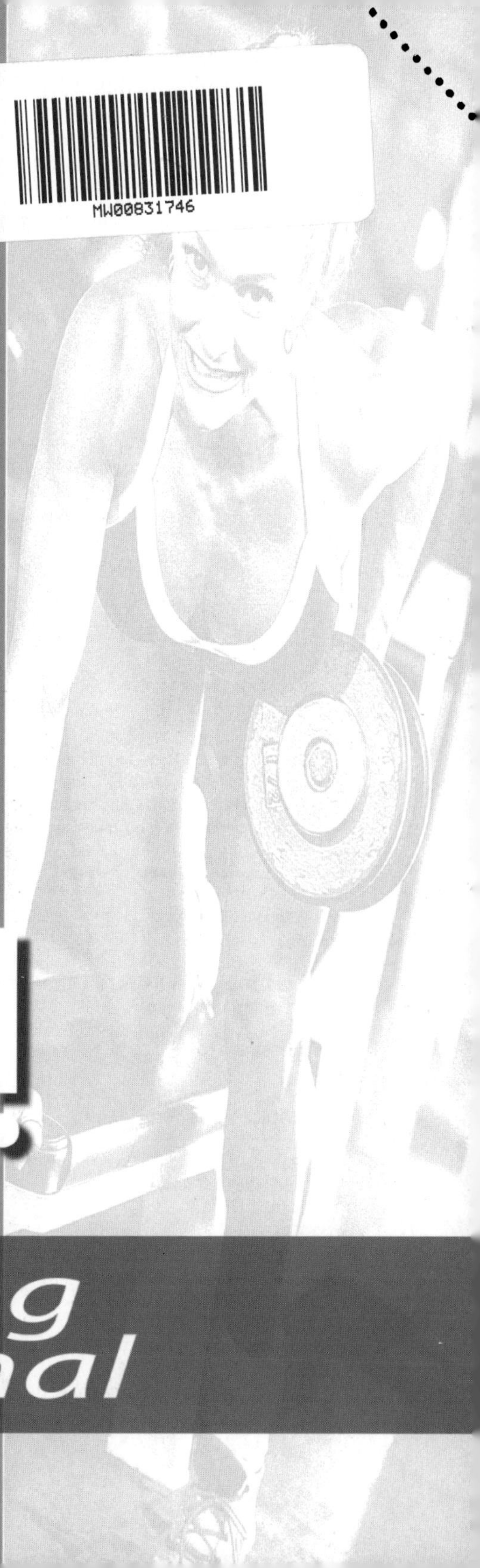

Published by MuscleMag International
5775 McLaughlin Road
Mississauga, ON Canada
L5R 3P7

Designed by Jackie Kydyk and Mandy Morgan
Written by Mandy Morgan

ISBN 1-55210-031-6

Distributed in Canada by
CANBOOK Distribution Services
c/o Pearson Canada
P.O. Box 335
195 Harry Walker Parkway N.
Newmarket, ON
L3Y 4X7

Distributed in the States by
BookWorld Services
1941 Whitfield Park Loop
Sarasota, FL 34243

Printed in Canada

Contributing Photographers
Alex Ardenti, Ralph DeHaan,
Irvin Gelb, Robert Kennedy,
Mike Kruckowski, Evan Klanfer,
Stewart Volland

General Information

Name: ______________________________

Address: ______________________________

City: ______________ State: __________ Zip: __________

Phone: ______________________________

Fax: ______________ Car: ______________

Company Name: ______________________________

Address: ______________________________

City: ______________ State: __________ Zip: __________

Phone: ______________________________

Fax: ______________________________

Emergency Information

Notify: ______________________________

Relationship: ______________________________

Phone: ______________ Work Phone: ______________

Address: ______________________________

City: ______________ State: __________ Zip: __________

Or Notify ______________ Relationship: ______________

Phone: ______________ Work Phone: ______________

Address: ______________ State: __________ Zip: __________

Medical Information

Physician: ______________ Phone: ______________

Insurance/HMO: ______________________________

Blood Type: ______________ Allergies: ______________

Automobile Information

Insurance Company: ______________________________

Policy Number: ______________________________

Drivers License Number: ______________________________

Expiry: ______________ Plate Number: ______________

Introduction

Taking your training seriously means recording your daily workouts, but such a task can be cumbersome and annoying. That's why *Oxygen* has put together a compact, organized training journal – it's all here – weight/set/rep charts, a heart-rate table for cardio, metric-conversion table to figure out your poundages, muscle-group illustrations for quick reference, a calendar for monthly goals and reminders, as well as a personal-data measurement table to access your weight and tape measurements over a 6-month period.

Easy-to-use and small enough not to be in the way while you're working out, *No Pain No Gain!* is the fitness enthusiast's ultimate companion.

Want to increase your poundages, decrease your bodyfat percentage, or work your abs, but don't remember what did the trick the last time? Here's your chance to easily record and reference your goals and the progress you make in achieving them. Find out which bodypart splits and training routines set you back or produce gains.

Reps, sets, training techniques – it's hard enough to remember what poundages you push from day to day, let alone month to month. So take advantage of this invaluable, in-your-face, tell-no-lies training journal for present and future reference. *No Pain No Gain!* – the ultimate companion.

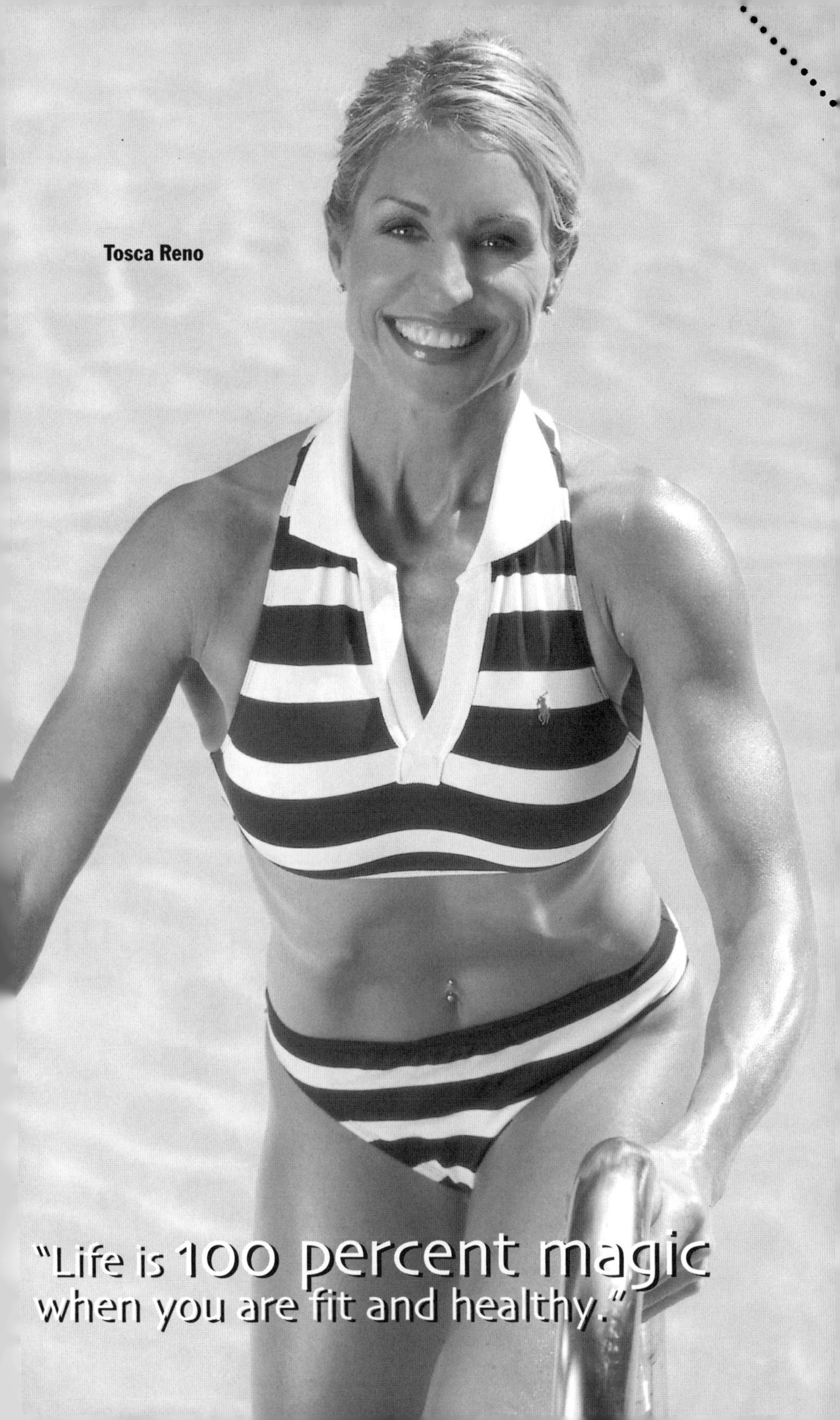
Tosca Reno
"Life is 100 percent magic
when you are fit and healthy."

Brandy Flores

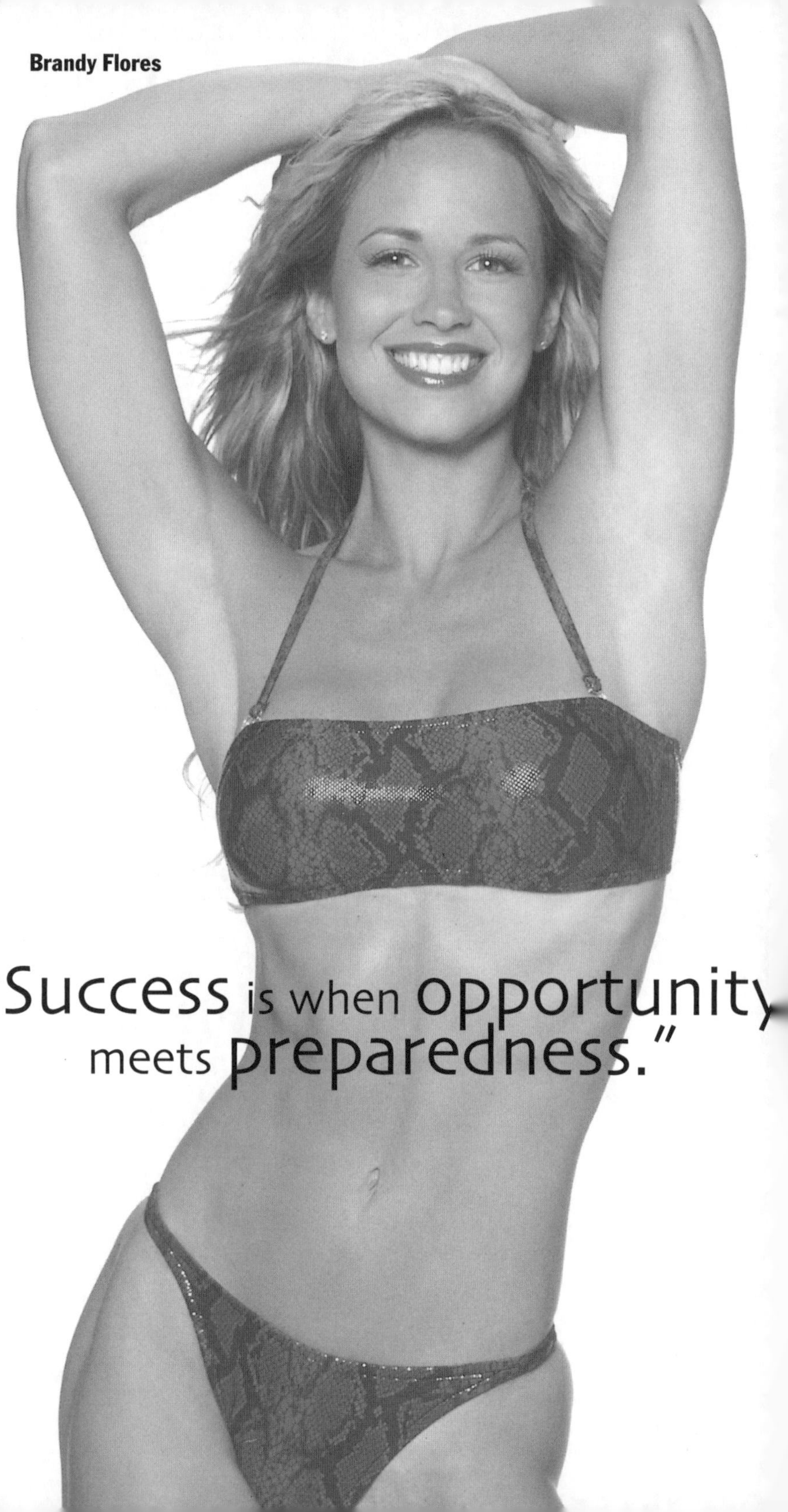

"Success is when opportunity meets preparedness."

DATE:	SET 1	SET 2	SET 3	SET 4	SET 5	SET 6	SET 7	SET 8
EXERCISE	WEIGHT	WEIGHT	WEIGHT	WEIGHT	WEIGHT	WEIGHT	WEIGHT	WEIGHT
	REPS	REPS	REPS	REPS	REPS	REPS	REPS	REPS

Cardio/Notes:

DATE:	SET 1	SET 2	SET 3	SET 4	SET 5	SET 6	SET 7	SET 8
EXERCISE	WEIGHT REPS	WEIGHT REPS	WEIGHT REPS	WEIGHT REPS	WEIGHT REPS	WEIGHT REPS	WEIGHT REPS	WEIGHT REPS

Cardio/Notes:

DATE:	SET 1	SET 2	SET 3	SET 4	SET 5	SET 6	SET 7	SET 8
EXERCISE	WEIGHT	WEIGHT	WEIGHT	WEIGHT	WEIGHT	WEIGHT	WEIGHT	WEIGHT
	REPS	REPS	REPS	REPS	REPS	REPS	REPS	REPS

Cardio/Notes:

DATE:	SET 1	SET 2	SET 3	SET 4	SET 5	SET 6	SET 7	SET 8
EXERCISE	WEIGHT	WEIGHT	WEIGHT	WEIGHT	WEIGHT	WEIGHT	WEIGHT	WEIGHT
	REPS	REPS	REPS	REPS	REPS	REPS	REPS	REPS

Cardio/Notes:

DATE:	SET 1	SET 2	SET 3	SET 4	SET 5	SET 6	SET 7	SET 8
EXERCISE	WEIGHT REPS	WEIGHT REPS	WEIGHT REPS	WEIGHT REPS	WEIGHT REPS	WEIGHT REPS	WEIGHT REPS	WEIGHT REPS

Cardio/Notes:

DATE:	SET 1	SET 2	SET 3	SET 4	SET 5	SET 6	SET 7	SET 8
EXERCISE	WEIGHT REPS	WEIGHT REPS	WEIGHT REPS	WEIGHT REPS	WEIGHT REPS	WEIGHT REPS	WEIGHT REPS	WEIGHT REPS

Cardio/Notes:

Visit www.oxygenmag.com

DATE:	SET 1	SET 2	SET 3	SET 4	SET 5	SET 6	SET 7	SET 8
EXERCISE	WEIGHT REPS	WEIGHT REPS	WEIGHT REPS	WEIGHT REPS	WEIGHT REPS	WEIGHT REPS	WEIGHT REPS	WEIGHT REPS

Cardio/Notes:

DATE:

EXERCISE	SET 1	SET 2	SET 3	SET 4	SET 5	SET 6	SET 7	SET 8
	WEIGHT REPS	WEIGHT REPS	WEIGHT REPS	WEIGHT REPS	WEIGHT REPS	WEIGHT REPS	WEIGHT REPS	WEIGHT REPS

Cardio/Notes:

DATE:	SET 1	SET 2	SET 3	SET 4	SET 5	SET 6	SET 7	SET 8
EXERCISE	WEIGHT	WEIGHT	WEIGHT	WEIGHT	WEIGHT	WEIGHT	WEIGHT	WEIGHT
	REPS	REPS	REPS	REPS	REPS	REPS	REPS	REPS

Cardio/Notes:

DATE:	SET 1	SET 2	SET 3	SET 4	SET 5	SET 6	SET 7	SET 8
EXERCISE	WEIGHT REPS	WEIGHT REPS	WEIGHT REPS	WEIGHT REPS	WEIGHT REPS	WEIGHT REPS	WEIGHT REPS	WEIGHT REPS

Cardio/Notes:

DATE:	SET 1	SET 2	SET 3	SET 4	SET 5	SET 6	SET 7	SET 8
EXERCISE	WEIGHT	WEIGHT	WEIGHT	WEIGHT	WEIGHT	WEIGHT	WEIGHT	WEIGHT
	REPS	REPS	REPS	REPS	REPS	REPS	REPS	REPS

Cardio/Notes:

DATE:	SET 1	SET 2	SET 3	SET 4	SET 5	SET 6	SET 7	SET 8
EXERCISE	WEIGHT	WEIGHT	WEIGHT	WEIGHT	WEIGHT	WEIGHT	WEIGHT	WEIGHT
	REPS	REPS	REPS	REPS	REPS	REPS	REPS	REPS

Cardio/Notes:

DATE:	SET 1	SET 2	SET 3	SET 4	SET 5	SET 6	SET 7	SET 8
EXERCISE	WEIGHT	WEIGHT	WEIGHT	WEIGHT	WEIGHT	WEIGHT	WEIGHT	WEIGHT
	REPS	REPS	REPS	REPS	REPS	REPS	REPS	REPS

Cardio/Notes:

DATE:

EXERCISE	SET 1	SET 2	SET 3	SET 4	SET 5	SET 6	SET 7	SET 8
	WEIGHT	WEIGHT	WEIGHT	WEIGHT	WEIGHT	WEIGHT	WEIGHT	WEIGHT
	REPS	REPS	REPS	REPS	REPS	REPS	REPS	REPS

Cardio/Notes:

DATE:	SET 1	SET 2	SET 3	SET 4	SET 5	SET 6	SET 7	SET 8
EXERCISE	WEIGHT REPS	WEIGHT REPS	WEIGHT REPS	WEIGHT REPS	WEIGHT REPS	WEIGHT REPS	WEIGHT REPS	WEIGHT REPS

Cardio/Notes:

DATE:	SET 1	SET 2	SET 3	SET 4	SET 5	SET 6	SET 7	SET 8
EXERCISE	WEIGHT	WEIGHT	WEIGHT	WEIGHT	WEIGHT	WEIGHT	WEIGHT	WEIGHT
	REPS	REPS	REPS	REPS	REPS	REPS	REPS	REPS

Cardio/Notes:

DATE:	SET 1	SET 2	SET 3	SET 4	SET 5	SET 6	SET 7	SET 8
EXERCISE	WEIGHT	WEIGHT	WEIGHT	WEIGHT	WEIGHT	WEIGHT	WEIGHT	WEIGHT
	REPS	REPS	REPS	REPS	REPS	REPS	REPS	REPS

Cardio/Notes:

DATE:	SET 1	SET 2	SET 3	SET 4	SET 5	SET 6	SET 7	SET 8
EXERCISE	WEIGHT REPS	WEIGHT REPS	WEIGHT REPS	WEIGHT REPS	WEIGHT REPS	WEIGHT REPS	WEIGHT REPS	WEIGHT REPS

Cardio/Notes:

DATE:	SET 1	SET 2	SET 3	SET 4	SET 5	SET 6	SET 7	SET 8
EXERCISE	WEIGHT	WEIGHT	WEIGHT	WEIGHT	WEIGHT	WEIGHT	WEIGHT	WEIGHT
	REPS	REPS	REPS	REPS	REPS	REPS	REPS	REPS

Cardio/Notes:

DATE:

EXERCISE	SET 1	SET 2	SET 3	SET 4	SET 5	SET 6	SET 7	SET 8
	WEIGHT	WEIGHT	WEIGHT	WEIGHT	WEIGHT	WEIGHT	WEIGHT	WEIGHT
	REPS	REPS	REPS	REPS	REPS	REPS	REPS	REPS

Cardio/Notes:

DATE:	SET 1	SET 2	SET 3	SET 4	SET 5	SET 6	SET 7	SET 8
EXERCISE	WEIGHT REPS	WEIGHT REPS	WEIGHT REPS	WEIGHT REPS	WEIGHT REPS	WEIGHT REPS	WEIGHT REPS	WEIGHT REPS

Cardio/Notes:

DATE:	SET 1	SET 2	SET 3	SET 4	SET 5	SET 6	SET 7	SET 8
EXERCISE	WEIGHT REPS	WEIGHT REPS	WEIGHT REPS	WEIGHT REPS	WEIGHT REPS	WEIGHT REPS	WEIGHT REPS	WEIGHT REPS

Cardio/Notes:

DATE:	SET 1	SET 2	SET 3	SET 4	SET 5	SET 6	SET 7	SET 8
EXERCISE	WEIGHT	WEIGHT	WEIGHT	WEIGHT	WEIGHT	WEIGHT	WEIGHT	WEIGHT
	REPS	REPS	REPS	REPS	REPS	REPS	REPS	REPS

Cardio/Notes:

DATE:	SET 1	SET 2	SET 3	SET 4	SET 5	SET 6	SET 7	SET 8
EXERCISE	WEIGHT REPS	WEIGHT REPS	WEIGHT REPS	WEIGHT REPS	WEIGHT REPS	WEIGHT REPS	WEIGHT REPS	WEIGHT REPS

Cardio/Notes:

DATE:	SET 1	SET 2	SET 3	SET 4	SET 5	SET 6	SET 7	SET 8
EXERCISE	WEIGHT	WEIGHT	WEIGHT	WEIGHT	WEIGHT	WEIGHT	WEIGHT	WEIGHT
	REPS	REPS	REPS	REPS	REPS	REPS	REPS	REPS

Cardio/Notes:

DATE:	SET 1	SET 2	SET 3	SET 4	SET 5	SET 6	SET 7	SET 8
EXERCISE	WEIGHT	WEIGHT	WEIGHT	WEIGHT	WEIGHT	WEIGHT	WEIGHT	WEIGHT
	REPS	REPS	REPS	REPS	REPS	REPS	REPS	REPS

Cardio/Notes:

DATE:	SET 1	SET 2	SET 3	SET 4	SET 5	SET 6	SET 7	SET 8
EXERCISE	WEIGHT	WEIGHT	WEIGHT	WEIGHT	WEIGHT	WEIGHT	WEIGHT	WEIGHT
	REPS	REPS	REPS	REPS	REPS	REPS	REPS	REPS

Cardio/Notes:

DATE:

EXERCISE	SET 1	SET 2	SET 3	SET 4	SET 5	SET 6	SET 7	SET 8
	WEIGHT	WEIGHT	WEIGHT	WEIGHT	WEIGHT	WEIGHT	WEIGHT	WEIGHT
	REPS	REPS	REPS	REPS	REPS	REPS	REPS	REPS

Cardio/Notes:

DATE:	SET 1	SET 2	SET 3	SET 4	SET 5	SET 6	SET 7	SET 8
EXERCISE	WEIGHT	WEIGHT	WEIGHT	WEIGHT	WEIGHT	WEIGHT	WEIGHT	WEIGHT
	REPS	REPS	REPS	REPS	REPS	REPS	REPS	REPS

Cardio/Notes:

DATE:	SET 1	SET 2	SET 3	SET 4	SET 5	SET 6	SET 7	SET 8
EXERCISE	WEIGHT	WEIGHT	WEIGHT	WEIGHT	WEIGHT	WEIGHT	WEIGHT	WEIGHT
	REPS	REPS	REPS	REPS	REPS	REPS	REPS	REPS

Cardio/Notes:

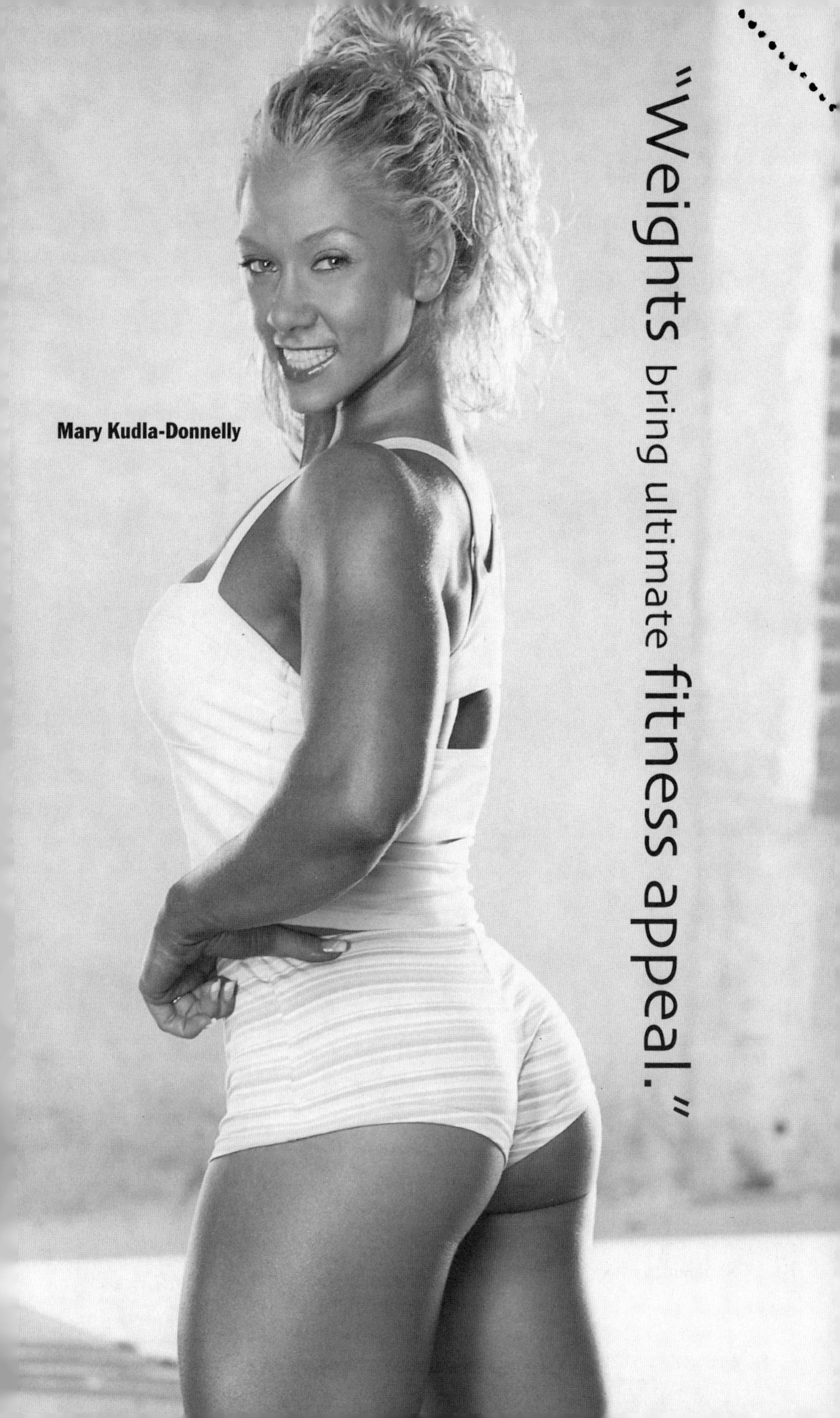

Mary Kudla-Donnelly

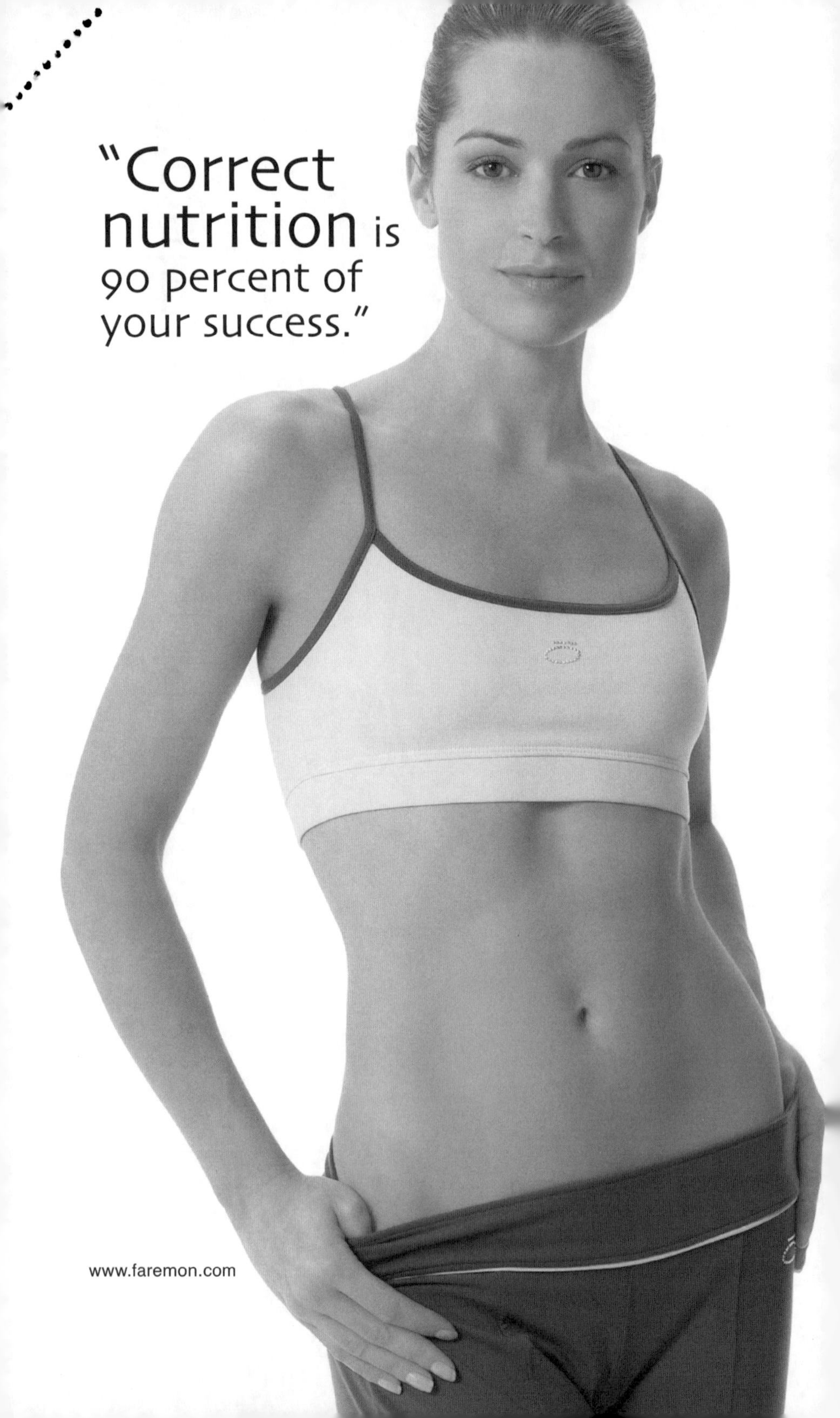
"Correct nutrition is 90 percent of your success."
www.faremon.com

DATE:	SET 1	SET 2	SET 3	SET 4	SET 5	SET 6	SET 7	SET 8
EXERCISE	WEIGHT REPS	WEIGHT REPS	WEIGHT REPS	WEIGHT REPS	WEIGHT REPS	WEIGHT REPS	WEIGHT REPS	WEIGHT REPS

Cardio/Notes:

DATE:

EXERCISE	SET 1	SET 2	SET 3	SET 4	SET 5	SET 6	SET 7	SET 8
	WEIGHT	WEIGHT	WEIGHT	WEIGHT	WEIGHT	WEIGHT	WEIGHT	WEIGHT
	REPS	REPS	REPS	REPS	REPS	REPS	REPS	REPS

Cardio/Notes:

DATE:	SET 1	SET 2	SET 3	SET 4	SET 5	SET 6	SET 7	SET 8
EXERCISE	WEIGHT REPS	WEIGHT REPS	WEIGHT REPS	WEIGHT REPS	WEIGHT REPS	WEIGHT REPS	WEIGHT REPS	WEIGHT REPS

Cardio/Notes:

DATE:	SET 1	SET 2	SET 3	SET 4	SET 5	SET 6	SET 7	SET 8
EXERCISE	WEIGHT REPS	WEIGHT REPS	WEIGHT REPS	WEIGHT REPS	WEIGHT REPS	WEIGHT REPS	WEIGHT REPS	WEIGHT REPS

Cardio/Notes:

DATE:	SET 1	SET 2	SET 3	SET 4	SET 5	SET 6	SET 7	SET 8
EXERCISE	WEIGHT	WEIGHT	WEIGHT	WEIGHT	WEIGHT	WEIGHT	WEIGHT	WEIGHT
	REPS	REPS	REPS	REPS	REPS	REPS	REPS	REPS

Cardio/Notes:

DATE:

EXERCISE	SET 1	SET 2	SET 3	SET 4	SET 5	SET 6	SET 7	SET 8
	WEIGHT	WEIGHT	WEIGHT	WEIGHT	WEIGHT	WEIGHT	WEIGHT	WEIGHT
	REPS	REPS	REPS	REPS	REPS	REPS	REPS	REPS

Cardio/Notes:

DATE:	SET 1	SET 2	SET 3	SET 4	SET 5	SET 6	SET 7	SET 8
EXERCISE	WEIGHT	WEIGHT	WEIGHT	WEIGHT	WEIGHT	WEIGHT	WEIGHT	WEIGHT
	REPS	REPS	REPS	REPS	REPS	REPS	REPS	REPS

Cardio/Notes:

DATE:

EXERCISE	SET 1	SET 2	SET 3	SET 4	SET 5	SET 6	SET 7	SET 8
	WEIGHT	WEIGHT	WEIGHT	WEIGHT	WEIGHT	WEIGHT	WEIGHT	WEIGHT
	REPS	REPS	REPS	REPS	REPS	REPS	REPS	REPS

Cardio/Notes:

DATE:	SET 1	SET 2	SET 3	SET 4	SET 5	SET 6	SET 7	SET 8
EXERCISE	WEIGHT	WEIGHT	WEIGHT	WEIGHT	WEIGHT	WEIGHT	WEIGHT	WEIGHT
	REPS	REPS	REPS	REPS	REPS	REPS	REPS	REPS

Cardio/Notes:

DATE:

EXERCISE	SET 1	SET 2	SET 3	SET 4	SET 5	SET 6	SET 7	SET 8
	WEIGHT / REPS	WEIGHT / REPS	WEIGHT / REPS	WEIGHT / REPS	WEIGHT / REPS	WEIGHT / REPS	WEIGHT / REPS	WEIGHT / REPS

Cardio/Notes:

DATE:	SET 1	SET 2	SET 3	SET 4	SET 5	SET 6	SET 7	SET 8
EXERCISE	WEIGHT	WEIGHT	WEIGHT	WEIGHT	WEIGHT	WEIGHT	WEIGHT	WEIGHT
	REPS	REPS	REPS	REPS	REPS	REPS	REPS	REPS

Cardio/Notes:

DATE:	SET 1	SET 2	SET 3	SET 4	SET 5	SET 6	SET 7	SET 8
EXERCISE	WEIGHT REPS	WEIGHT REPS	WEIGHT REPS	WEIGHT REPS	WEIGHT REPS	WEIGHT REPS	WEIGHT REPS	WEIGHT REPS

Cardio/Notes:

DATE:	SET 1	SET 2	SET 3	SET 4	SET 5	SET 6	SET 7	SET 8
EXERCISE	WEIGHT	WEIGHT	WEIGHT	WEIGHT	WEIGHT	WEIGHT	WEIGHT	WEIGHT
	REPS	REPS	REPS	REPS	REPS	REPS	REPS	REPS

Cardio/Notes:

DATE:

EXERCISE	SET 1	SET 2	SET 3	SET 4	SET 5	SET 6	SET 7	SET 8
	WEIGHT / REPS	WEIGHT / REPS	WEIGHT / REPS	WEIGHT / REPS	WEIGHT / REPS	WEIGHT / REPS	WEIGHT / REPS	WEIGHT / REPS

Cardio/Notes:

DATE:	SET 1	SET 2	SET 3	SET 4	SET 5	SET 6	SET 7	SET 8
EXERCISE	WEIGHT	WEIGHT	WEIGHT	WEIGHT	WEIGHT	WEIGHT	WEIGHT	WEIGHT
	REPS	REPS	REPS	REPS	REPS	REPS	REPS	REPS

Cardio/Notes:

DATE:	SET 1	SET 2	SET 3	SET 4	SET 5	SET 6	SET 7	SET 8
EXERCISE	WEIGHT	WEIGHT	WEIGHT	WEIGHT	WEIGHT	WEIGHT	WEIGHT	WEIGHT
	REPS	REPS	REPS	REPS	REPS	REPS	REPS	REPS

Cardio/Notes:

DATE:	SET 1	SET 2	SET 3	SET 4	SET 5	SET 6	SET 7	SET 8
EXERCISE	WEIGHT REPS	WEIGHT REPS	WEIGHT REPS	WEIGHT REPS	WEIGHT REPS	WEIGHT REPS	WEIGHT REPS	WEIGHT REPS

Cardio/Notes:

DATE:	SET 1	SET 2	SET 3	SET 4	SET 5	SET 6	SET 7	SET 8
EXERCISE	WEIGHT REPS	WEIGHT REPS	WEIGHT REPS	WEIGHT REPS	WEIGHT REPS	WEIGHT REPS	WEIGHT REPS	WEIGHT REPS

Cardio/Notes:

DATE:	SET 1	SET 2	SET 3	SET 4	SET 5	SET 6	SET 7	SET 8
EXERCISE	WEIGHT	WEIGHT	WEIGHT	WEIGHT	WEIGHT	WEIGHT	WEIGHT	WEIGHT
	REPS	REPS	REPS	REPS	REPS	REPS	REPS	REPS

Cardio/Notes:

DATE:	SET 1	SET 2	SET 3	SET 4	SET 5	SET 6	SET 7	SET 8
EXERCISE	WEIGHT	WEIGHT	WEIGHT	WEIGHT	WEIGHT	WEIGHT	WEIGHT	WEIGHT
	REPS	REPS	REPS	REPS	REPS	REPS	REPS	REPS

Cardio/Notes:

DATE:	SET 1	SET 2	SET 3	SET 4	SET 5	SET 6	SET 7	SET 8
EXERCISE	WEIGHT	WEIGHT	WEIGHT	WEIGHT	WEIGHT	WEIGHT	WEIGHT	WEIGHT
	REPS	REPS	REPS	REPS	REPS	REPS	REPS	REPS

Cardio/Notes:

DATE:	SET 1	SET 2	SET 3	SET 4	SET 5	SET 6	SET 7	SET 8
EXERCISE	WEIGHT	WEIGHT	WEIGHT	WEIGHT	WEIGHT	WEIGHT	WEIGHT	WEIGHT
	REPS	REPS	REPS	REPS	REPS	REPS	REPS	REPS

Cardio/Notes:

DATE:	SET 1	SET 2	SET 3	SET 4	SET 5	SET 6	SET 7	SET 8
EXERCISE	WEIGHT	WEIGHT	WEIGHT	WEIGHT	WEIGHT	WEIGHT	WEIGHT	WEIGHT
	REPS	REPS	REPS	REPS	REPS	REPS	REPS	REPS

Cardio/Notes:

DATE:

EXERCISE	SET 1	SET 2	SET 3	SET 4	SET 5	SET 6	SET 7	SET 8
	WEIGHT	WEIGHT	WEIGHT	WEIGHT	WEIGHT	WEIGHT	WEIGHT	WEIGHT
	REPS	REPS	REPS	REPS	REPS	REPS	REPS	REPS

Cardio/Notes:

DATE:	SET 1	SET 2	SET 3	SET 4	SET 5	SET 6	SET 7	SET 8
EXERCISE	WEIGHT	WEIGHT	WEIGHT	WEIGHT	WEIGHT	WEIGHT	WEIGHT	WEIGHT
	REPS	REPS	REPS	REPS	REPS	REPS	REPS	REPS

Cardio/Notes:

DATE:	SET 1	SET 2	SET 3	SET 4	SET 5	SET 6	SET 7	SET 8
EXERCISE	WEIGHT	WEIGHT	WEIGHT	WEIGHT	WEIGHT	WEIGHT	WEIGHT	WEIGHT
	REPS	REPS	REPS	REPS	REPS	REPS	REPS	REPS

Cardio/Notes:

DATE:	SET 1	SET 2	SET 3	SET 4	SET 5	SET 6	SET 7	SET 8
EXERCISE	WEIGHT REPS	WEIGHT REPS	WEIGHT REPS	WEIGHT REPS	WEIGHT REPS	WEIGHT REPS	WEIGHT REPS	WEIGHT REPS

Cardio/Notes:

DATE:	SET 1	SET 2	SET 3	SET 4	SET 5	SET 6	SET 7	SET 8
EXERCISE	WEIGHT REPS	WEIGHT REPS	WEIGHT REPS	WEIGHT REPS	WEIGHT REPS	WEIGHT REPS	WEIGHT REPS	WEIGHT REPS

Cardio/Notes:

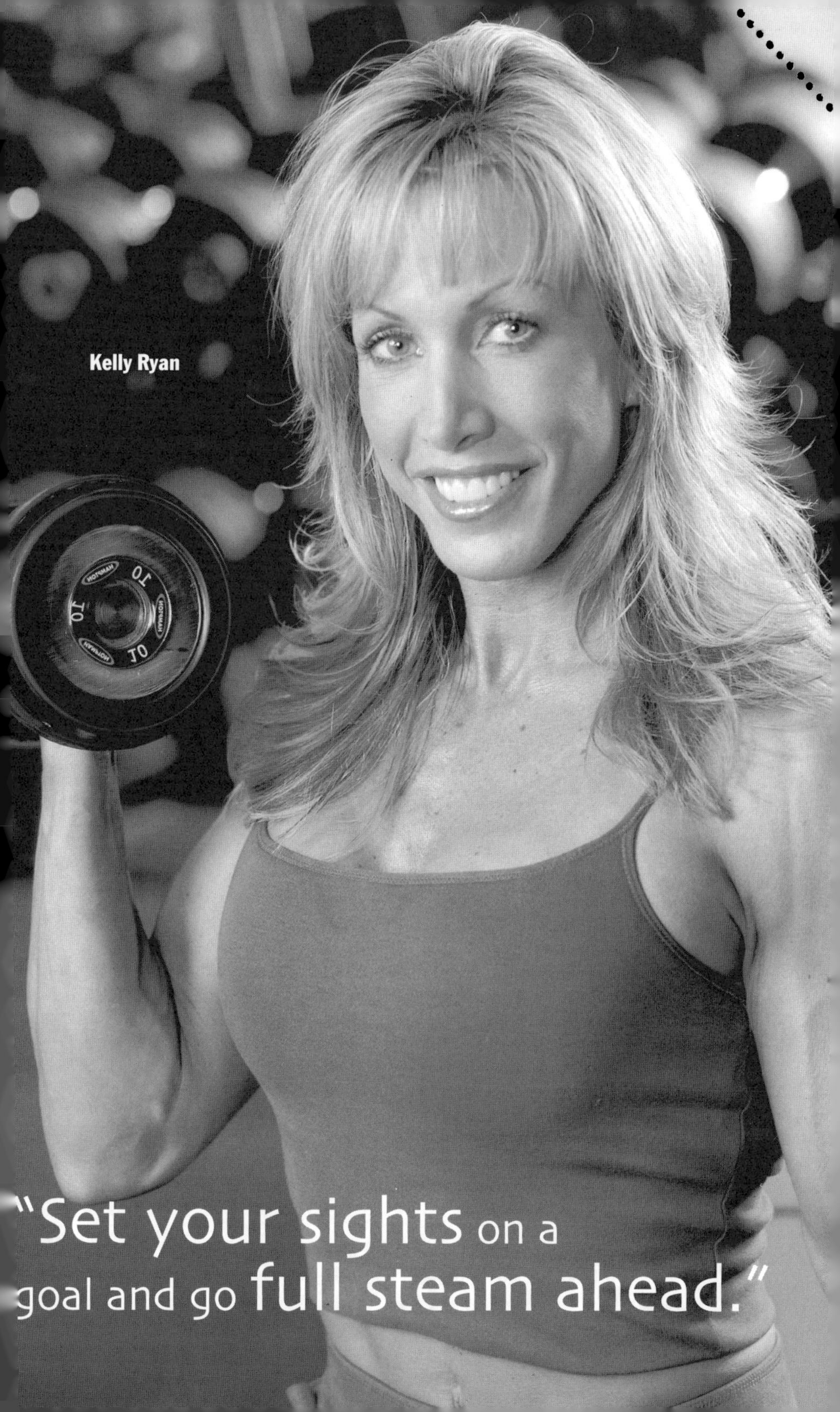
Kelly Ryan
"Set your sights on a goal and go full steam ahead."

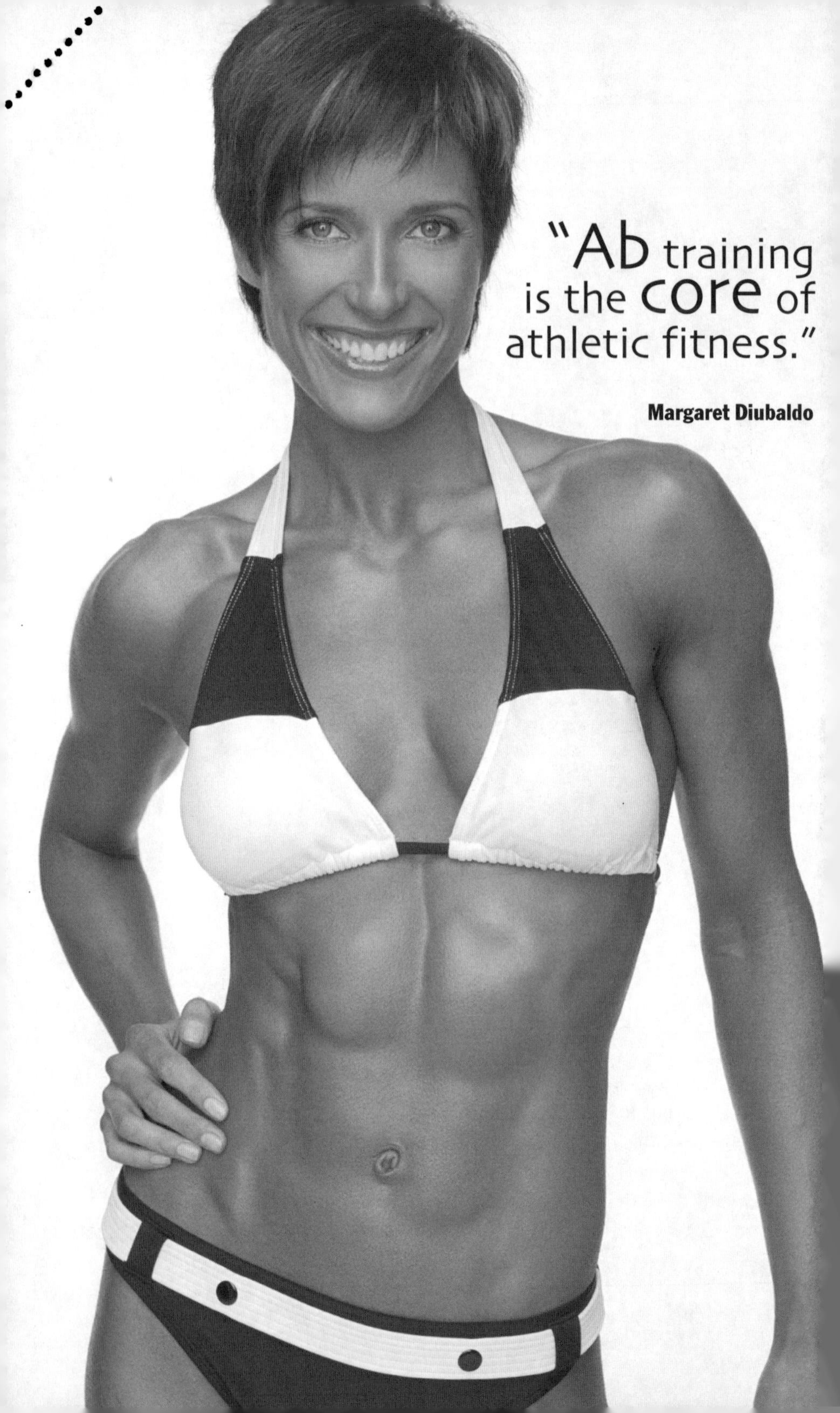

"Ab training is the core of athletic fitness."

Margaret Diubaldo

DATE:

EXERCISE	SET 1	SET 2	SET 3	SET 4	SET 5	SET 6	SET 7	SET 8
	WEIGHT REPS	WEIGHT REPS	WEIGHT REPS	WEIGHT REPS	WEIGHT REPS	WEIGHT REPS	WEIGHT REPS	WEIGHT REPS

Cardio/Notes:

DATE:

EXERCISE	SET 1	SET 2	SET 3	SET 4	SET 5	SET 6	SET 7	SET 8
	WEIGHT	WEIGHT	WEIGHT	WEIGHT	WEIGHT	WEIGHT	WEIGHT	WEIGHT
	REPS	REPS	REPS	REPS	REPS	REPS	REPS	REPS

Cardio/Notes:

DATE:	SET 1	SET 2	SET 3	SET 4	SET 5	SET 6	SET 7	SET 8
EXERCISE	WEIGHT	WEIGHT	WEIGHT	WEIGHT	WEIGHT	WEIGHT	WEIGHT	WEIGHT
	REPS	REPS	REPS	REPS	REPS	REPS	REPS	REPS

Cardio/Notes:

DATE:	SET 1	SET 2	SET 3	SET 4	SET 5	SET 6	SET 7	SET 8
EXERCISE	WEIGHT	WEIGHT	WEIGHT	WEIGHT	WEIGHT	WEIGHT	WEIGHT	WEIGHT
	REPS	REPS	REPS	REPS	REPS	REPS	REPS	REPS

Cardio/Notes:

DATE:	SET 1	SET 2	SET 3	SET 4	SET 5	SET 6	SET 7	SET 8
EXERCISE	WEIGHT	WEIGHT	WEIGHT	WEIGHT	WEIGHT	WEIGHT	WEIGHT	WEIGHT
	REPS	REPS	REPS	REPS	REPS	REPS	REPS	REPS

Cardio/Notes:

DATE:	SET 1	SET 2	SET 3	SET 4	SET 5	SET 6	SET 7	SET 8
EXERCISE	WEIGHT	WEIGHT	WEIGHT	WEIGHT	WEIGHT	WEIGHT	WEIGHT	WEIGHT
	REPS	REPS	REPS	REPS	REPS	REPS	REPS	REPS

Cardio/Notes:

DATE:	SET 1	SET 2	SET 3	SET 4	SET 5	SET 6	SET 7	SET 8
EXERCISE	WEIGHT REPS	WEIGHT REPS	WEIGHT REPS	WEIGHT REPS	WEIGHT REPS	WEIGHT REPS	WEIGHT REPS	WEIGHT REPS

Cardio/Notes:

DATE:	SET 1	SET 2	SET 3	SET 4	SET 5	SET 6	SET 7	SET 8
EXERCISE	WEIGHT	WEIGHT	WEIGHT	WEIGHT	WEIGHT	WEIGHT	WEIGHT	WEIGHT
	REPS	REPS	REPS	REPS	REPS	REPS	REPS	REPS

Cardio/Notes:

DATE:	SET 1	SET 2	SET 3	SET 4	SET 5	SET 6	SET 7	SET 8
EXERCISE	WEIGHT	WEIGHT	WEIGHT	WEIGHT	WEIGHT	WEIGHT	WEIGHT	WEIGHT
	REPS	REPS	REPS	REPS	REPS	REPS	REPS	REPS

Cardio/Notes:

DATE:

EXERCISE	SET 1	SET 2	SET 3	SET 4	SET 5	SET 6	SET 7	SET 8
	WEIGHT REPS	WEIGHT REPS	WEIGHT REPS	WEIGHT REPS	WEIGHT REPS	WEIGHT REPS	WEIGHT REPS	WEIGHT REPS

Cardio/Notes:

DATE:	SET 1	SET 2	SET 3	SET 4	SET 5	SET 6	SET 7	SET 8
EXERCISE	WEIGHT	WEIGHT	WEIGHT	WEIGHT	WEIGHT	WEIGHT	WEIGHT	WEIGHT
	REPS	REPS	REPS	REPS	REPS	REPS	REPS	REPS

Cardio/Notes:

DATE:	SET 1	SET 2	SET 3	SET 4	SET 5	SET 6	SET 7	SET 8
EXERCISE	WEIGHT	WEIGHT	WEIGHT	WEIGHT	WEIGHT	WEIGHT	WEIGHT	WEIGHT
	REPS	REPS	REPS	REPS	REPS	REPS	REPS	REPS

Cardio/Notes:

DATE:	SET 1	SET 2	SET 3	SET 4	SET 5	SET 6	SET 7	SET 8
EXERCISE	WEIGHT REPS	WEIGHT REPS	WEIGHT REPS	WEIGHT REPS	WEIGHT REPS	WEIGHT REPS	WEIGHT REPS	WEIGHT REPS

Cardio/Notes:

DATE:

EXERCISE	SET 1	SET 2	SET 3	SET 4	SET 5	SET 6	SET 7	SET 8
	WEIGHT	WEIGHT	WEIGHT	WEIGHT	WEIGHT	WEIGHT	WEIGHT	WEIGHT
	REPS	REPS	REPS	REPS	REPS	REPS	REPS	REPS

Cardio/Notes:

DATE:	SET 1	SET 2	SET 3	SET 4	SET 5	SET 6	SET 7	SET 8
EXERCISE	WEIGHT	WEIGHT	WEIGHT	WEIGHT	WEIGHT	WEIGHT	WEIGHT	WEIGHT
	REPS	REPS	REPS	REPS	REPS	REPS	REPS	REPS

Cardio/Notes:

DATE:	SET 1	SET 2	SET 3	SET 4	SET 5	SET 6	SET 7	SET 8
EXERCISE	WEIGHT	WEIGHT	WEIGHT	WEIGHT	WEIGHT	WEIGHT	WEIGHT	WEIGHT
	REPS	REPS	REPS	REPS	REPS	REPS	REPS	REPS

Cardio/Notes:

DATE:	SET 1	SET 2	SET 3	SET 4	SET 5	SET 6	SET 7	SET 8
EXERCISE	WEIGHT REPS	WEIGHT REPS	WEIGHT REPS	WEIGHT REPS	WEIGHT REPS	WEIGHT REPS	WEIGHT REPS	WEIGHT REPS

Cardio/Notes:

DATE:	SET 1	SET 2	SET 3	SET 4	SET 5	SET 6	SET 7	SET 8
EXERCISE	WEIGHT	WEIGHT	WEIGHT	WEIGHT	WEIGHT	WEIGHT	WEIGHT	WEIGHT
	REPS	REPS	REPS	REPS	REPS	REPS	REPS	REPS

Cardio/Notes:

DATE:	SET 1	SET 2	SET 3	SET 4	SET 5	SET 6	SET 7	SET 8
EXERCISE	WEIGHT	WEIGHT	WEIGHT	WEIGHT	WEIGHT	WEIGHT	WEIGHT	WEIGHT
	REPS	REPS	REPS	REPS	REPS	REPS	REPS	REPS

Cardio/Notes:

DATE:	SET 1	SET 2	SET 3	SET 4	SET 5	SET 6	SET 7	SET 8
EXERCISE	WEIGHT REPS	WEIGHT REPS	WEIGHT REPS	WEIGHT REPS	WEIGHT REPS	WEIGHT REPS	WEIGHT REPS	WEIGHT REPS

Cardio/Notes:

DATE:	SET 1	SET 2	SET 3	SET 4	SET 5	SET 6	SET 7	SET 8
EXERCISE	WEIGHT	WEIGHT	WEIGHT	WEIGHT	WEIGHT	WEIGHT	WEIGHT	WEIGHT
	REPS	REPS	REPS	REPS	REPS	REPS	REPS	REPS

Cardio/Notes:

DATE:	SET 1	SET 2	SET 3	SET 4	SET 5	SET 6	SET 7	SET 8
EXERCISE	WEIGHT	WEIGHT	WEIGHT	WEIGHT	WEIGHT	WEIGHT	WEIGHT	WEIGHT
	REPS	REPS	REPS	REPS	REPS	REPS	REPS	REPS

Cardio/Notes:

DATE:	SET 1	SET 2	SET 3	SET 4	SET 5	SET 6	SET 7	SET 8
EXERCISE	WEIGHT	WEIGHT	WEIGHT	WEIGHT	WEIGHT	WEIGHT	WEIGHT	WEIGHT
	REPS	REPS	REPS	REPS	REPS	REPS	REPS	REPS

Cardio/Notes:

DATE:	SET 1	SET 2	SET 3	SET 4	SET 5	SET 6	SET 7	SET 8
EXERCISE	WEIGHT	WEIGHT	WEIGHT	WEIGHT	WEIGHT	WEIGHT	WEIGHT	WEIGHT
	REPS	REPS	REPS	REPS	REPS	REPS	REPS	REPS

Cardio/Notes:

DATE:	SET 1	SET 2	SET 3	SET 4	SET 5	SET 6	SET 7	SET 8
EXERCISE	WEIGHT REPS	WEIGHT REPS	WEIGHT REPS	WEIGHT REPS	WEIGHT REPS	WEIGHT REPS	WEIGHT REPS	WEIGHT REPS

Cardio/Notes:

DATE:	SET 1	SET 2	SET 3	SET 4	SET 5	SET 6	SET 7	SET 8
EXERCISE	WEIGHT	WEIGHT	WEIGHT	WEIGHT	WEIGHT	WEIGHT	WEIGHT	WEIGHT
	REPS	REPS	REPS	REPS	REPS	REPS	REPS	REPS

Cardio/Notes:

DATE:	SET 1	SET 2	SET 3	SET 4	SET 5	SET 6	SET 7	SET 8
EXERCISE	WEIGHT REPS	WEIGHT REPS	WEIGHT REPS	WEIGHT REPS	WEIGHT REPS	WEIGHT REPS	WEIGHT REPS	WEIGHT REPS

Cardio/Notes:

DATE:	SET 1	SET 2	SET 3	SET 4	SET 5	SET 6	SET 7	SET 8
EXERCISE	WEIGHT REPS	WEIGHT REPS	WEIGHT REPS	WEIGHT REPS	WEIGHT REPS	WEIGHT REPS	WEIGHT REPS	WEIGHT REPS

Cardio/Notes:

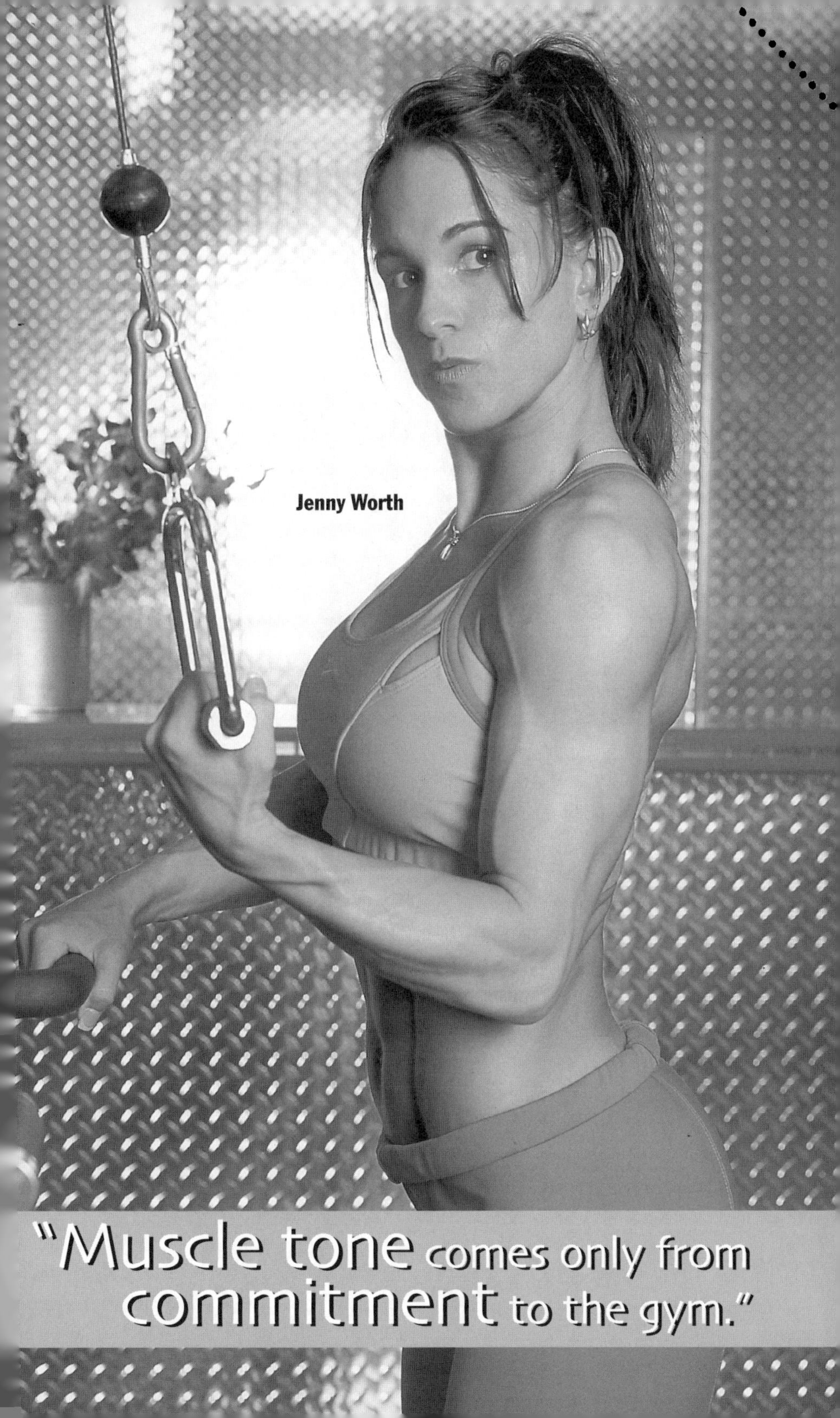

Jenny Worth

"Muscle tone comes only from commitment to the gym."

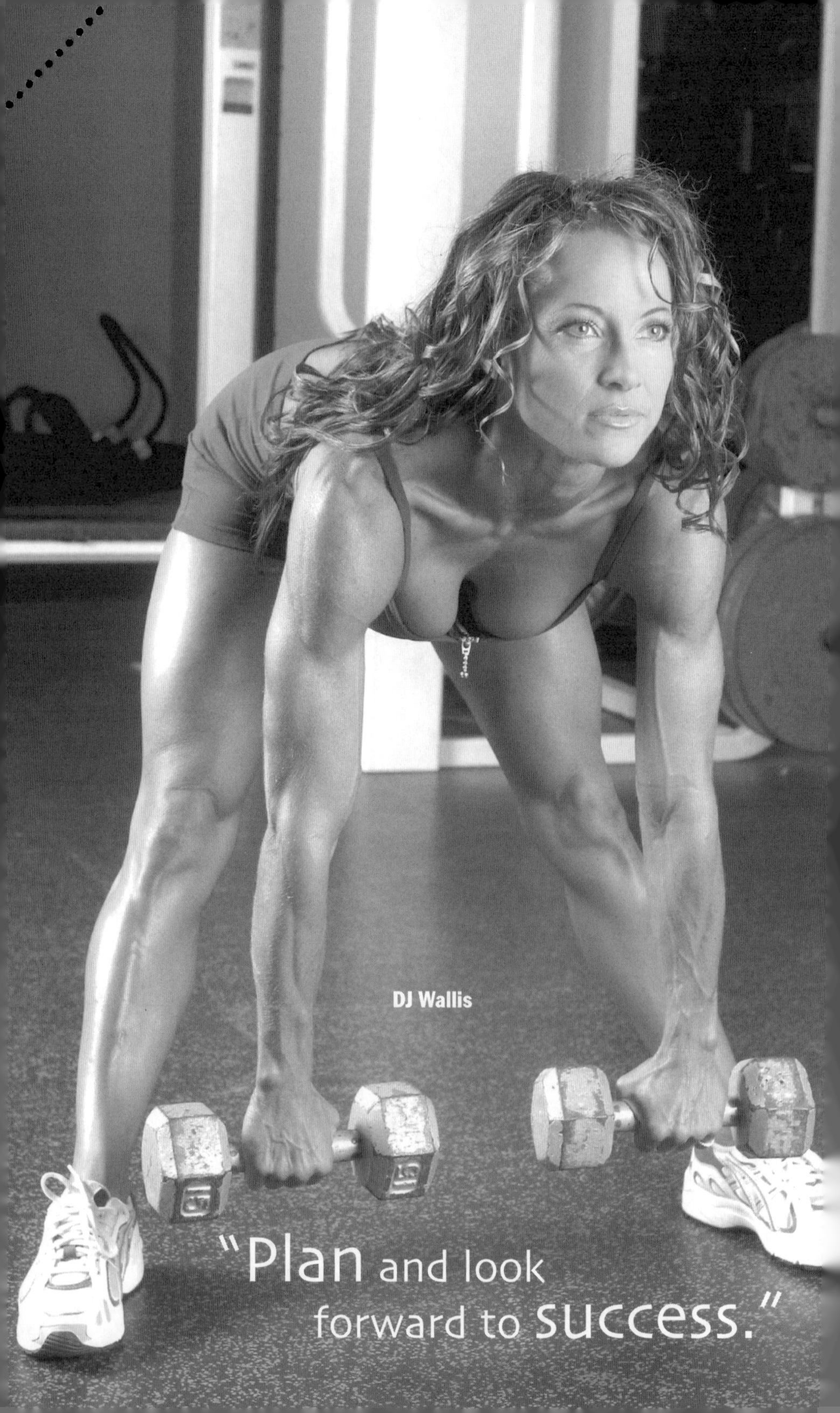

DJ Wallis

"Plan and look forward to success."

DATE:	SET 1	SET 2	SET 3	SET 4	SET 5	SET 6	SET 7	SET 8
EXERCISE	WEIGHT	WEIGHT	WEIGHT	WEIGHT	WEIGHT	WEIGHT	WEIGHT	WEIGHT
	REPS	REPS	REPS	REPS	REPS	REPS	REPS	REPS

Cardio/Notes:

DATE:	SET 1	SET 2	SET 3	SET 4	SET 5	SET 6	SET 7	SET 8
EXERCISE	WEIGHT REPS	WEIGHT REPS	WEIGHT REPS	WEIGHT REPS	WEIGHT REPS	WEIGHT REPS	WEIGHT REPS	WEIGHT REPS

Cardio/Notes:

DATE:	SET 1	SET 2	SET 3	SET 4	SET 5	SET 6	SET 7	SET 8
EXERCISE	WEIGHT REPS	WEIGHT REPS	WEIGHT REPS	WEIGHT REPS	WEIGHT REPS	WEIGHT REPS	WEIGHT REPS	WEIGHT REPS

Cardio/Notes:

DATE:

EXERCISE	SET 1	SET 2	SET 3	SET 4	SET 5	SET 6	SET 7	SET 8
	WEIGHT / REPS	WEIGHT / REPS	WEIGHT / REPS	WEIGHT / REPS	WEIGHT / REPS	WEIGHT / REPS	WEIGHT / REPS	WEIGHT / REPS

Cardio/Notes:

DATE:	SET 1	SET 2	SET 3	SET 4	SET 5	SET 6	SET 7	SET 8
EXERCISE	WEIGHT	WEIGHT	WEIGHT	WEIGHT	WEIGHT	WEIGHT	WEIGHT	WEIGHT
	REPS	REPS	REPS	REPS	REPS	REPS	REPS	REPS

Cardio/Notes:

DATE:

EXERCISE	SET 1	SET 2	SET 3	SET 4	SET 5	SET 6	SET 7	SET 8
	WEIGHT REPS	WEIGHT REPS	WEIGHT REPS	WEIGHT REPS	WEIGHT REPS	WEIGHT REPS	WEIGHT REPS	WEIGHT REPS

Cardio/Notes:

DATE:	SET 1	SET 2	SET 3	SET 4	SET 5	SET 6	SET 7	SET 8
EXERCISE	WEIGHT	WEIGHT	WEIGHT	WEIGHT	WEIGHT	WEIGHT	WEIGHT	WEIGHT
	REPS	REPS	REPS	REPS	REPS	REPS	REPS	REPS

Cardio/Notes:

DATE:	SET 1	SET 2	SET 3	SET 4	SET 5	SET 6	SET 7	SET 8
EXERCISE	WEIGHT	WEIGHT	WEIGHT	WEIGHT	WEIGHT	WEIGHT	WEIGHT	WEIGHT
	REPS	REPS	REPS	REPS	REPS	REPS	REPS	REPS

Cardio/Notes:

DATE:	SET 1	SET 2	SET 3	SET 4	SET 5	SET 6	SET 7	SET 8
EXERCISE	WEIGHT	WEIGHT	WEIGHT	WEIGHT	WEIGHT	WEIGHT	WEIGHT	WEIGHT
	REPS	REPS	REPS	REPS	REPS	REPS	REPS	REPS

Cardio/Notes:

DATE:	SET 1	SET 2	SET 3	SET 4	SET 5	SET 6	SET 7	SET 8
EXERCISE	WEIGHT	WEIGHT	WEIGHT	WEIGHT	WEIGHT	WEIGHT	WEIGHT	WEIGHT
	REPS	REPS	REPS	REPS	REPS	REPS	REPS	REPS

Cardio/Notes:

DATE:	SET 1	SET 2	SET 3	SET 4	SET 5	SET 6	SET 7	SET 8
EXERCISE	WEIGHT REPS	WEIGHT REPS	WEIGHT REPS	WEIGHT REPS	WEIGHT REPS	WEIGHT REPS	WEIGHT REPS	WEIGHT REPS

Cardio/Notes:

DATE:

EXERCISE	SET 1	SET 2	SET 3	SET 4	SET 5	SET 6	SET 7	SET 8
	WEIGHT REPS	WEIGHT REPS	WEIGHT REPS	WEIGHT REPS	WEIGHT REPS	WEIGHT REPS	WEIGHT REPS	WEIGHT REPS

Cardio/Notes:

DATE:	SET 1	SET 2	SET 3	SET 4	SET 5	SET 6	SET 7	SET 8
EXERCISE	WEIGHT	WEIGHT	WEIGHT	WEIGHT	WEIGHT	WEIGHT	WEIGHT	WEIGHT
	REPS	REPS	REPS	REPS	REPS	REPS	REPS	REPS

Cardio/Notes:

DATE:

EXERCISE	SET 1	SET 2	SET 3	SET 4	SET 5	SET 6	SET 7	SET 8
	WEIGHT	WEIGHT	WEIGHT	WEIGHT	WEIGHT	WEIGHT	WEIGHT	WEIGHT
	REPS	REPS	REPS	REPS	REPS	REPS	REPS	REPS

Cardio/Notes:

DATE:	SET 1	SET 2	SET 3	SET 4	SET 5	SET 6	SET 7	SET 8
EXERCISE	WEIGHT	WEIGHT	WEIGHT	WEIGHT	WEIGHT	WEIGHT	WEIGHT	WEIGHT
	REPS	REPS	REPS	REPS	REPS	REPS	REPS	REPS

Cardio/Notes:

DATE:	SET 1	SET 2	SET 3	SET 4	SET 5	SET 6	SET 7	SET 8
EXERCISE	WEIGHT REPS	WEIGHT REPS	WEIGHT REPS	WEIGHT REPS	WEIGHT REPS	WEIGHT REPS	WEIGHT REPS	WEIGHT REPS

Cardio/Notes:

DATE:

	SET 1	SET 2	SET 3	SET 4	SET 5	SET 6	SET 7	SET 8
EXERCISE	WEIGHT	WEIGHT	WEIGHT	WEIGHT	WEIGHT	WEIGHT	WEIGHT	WEIGHT
	REPS	REPS	REPS	REPS	REPS	REPS	REPS	REPS

ardio/Notes:

DATE:	SET 1	SET 2	SET 3	SET 4	SET 5	SET 6	SET 7	SET 8
EXERCISE	WEIGHT	WEIGHT	WEIGHT	WEIGHT	WEIGHT	WEIGHT	WEIGHT	WEIGH
	REPS	REPS	REPS	REPS	REPS	REPS	REPS	REPS

Cardio/Notes:

DATE:	SET 1	SET 2	SET 3	SET 4	SET 5	SET 6	SET 7	SET 8
EXERCISE	WEIGHT	WEIGHT	WEIGHT	WEIGHT	WEIGHT	WEIGHT	WEIGHT	WEIGHT
	REPS	REPS	REPS	REPS	REPS	REPS	REPS	REPS

Cardio/Notes:

DATE:

EXERCISE	SET 1	SET 2	SET 3	SET 4	SET 5	SET 6	SET 7	SET 8
	WEIGHT	WEIGHT	WEIGHT	WEIGHT	WEIGHT	WEIGHT	WEIGHT	WEIGHT
	REPS	REPS	REPS	REPS	REPS	REPS	REPS	REPS

Cardio/Notes:

DATE:	SET 1	SET 2	SET 3	SET 4	SET 5	SET 6	SET 7	SET 8
EXERCISE	WEIGHT	WEIGHT	WEIGHT	WEIGHT	WEIGHT	WEIGHT	WEIGHT	WEIGHT
	REPS	REPS	REPS	REPS	REPS	REPS	REPS	REPS

Cardio/Notes:

DATE:

EXERCISE	SET 1	SET 2	SET 3	SET 4	SET 5	SET 6	SET 7	SET 8
	WEIGHT	WEIGHT	WEIGHT	WEIGHT	WEIGHT	WEIGHT	WEIGHT	WEIGHT
	REPS	REPS	REPS	REPS	REPS	REPS	REPS	REPS

Cardio/Notes:

DATE:	SET 1	SET 2	SET 3	SET 4	SET 5	SET 6	SET 7	SET 8
EXERCISE	WEIGHT REPS	WEIGHT REPS	WEIGHT REPS	WEIGHT REPS	WEIGHT REPS	WEIGHT REPS	WEIGHT REPS	WEIGHT REPS

Cardio/Notes:

DATE:	SET 1	SET 2	SET 3	SET 4	SET 5	SET 6	SET 7	SET 8
EXERCISE	WEIGHT	WEIGHT	WEIGHT	WEIGHT	WEIGHT	WEIGHT	WEIGHT	WEIGHT
	REPS	REPS	REPS	REPS	REPS	REPS	REPS	REPS

Cardio/Notes:

DATE:	SET 1	SET 2	SET 3	SET 4	SET 5	SET 6	SET 7	SET 8
EXERCISE	WEIGHT REPS	WEIGHT REPS	WEIGHT REPS	WEIGHT REPS	WEIGHT REPS	WEIGHT REPS	WEIGHT REPS	WEIGHT REPS

Cardio/Notes:

DATE:

EXERCISE	SET 1	SET 2	SET 3	SET 4	SET 5	SET 6	SET 7	SET 8
	WEIGHT	WEIGHT	WEIGHT	WEIGHT	WEIGHT	WEIGHT	WEIGHT	WEIGHT
	REPS	REPS	REPS	REPS	REPS	REPS	REPS	REPS

Cardio/Notes:

DATE:	SET 1	SET 2	SET 3	SET 4	SET 5	SET 6	SET 7	SET 8
EXERCISE	WEIGHT	WEIGHT	WEIGHT	WEIGHT	WEIGHT	WEIGHT	WEIGHT	WEIGHT
	REPS	REPS	REPS	REPS	REPS	REPS	REPS	REPS

Cardio/Notes:

DATE:	SET 1	SET 2	SET 3	SET 4	SET 5	SET 6	SET 7	SET 8
EXERCISE	WEIGHT	WEIGHT	WEIGHT	WEIGHT	WEIGHT	WEIGHT	WEIGHT	WEIGHT
	REPS	REPS	REPS	REPS	REPS	REPS	REPS	REPS

Cardio/Notes:

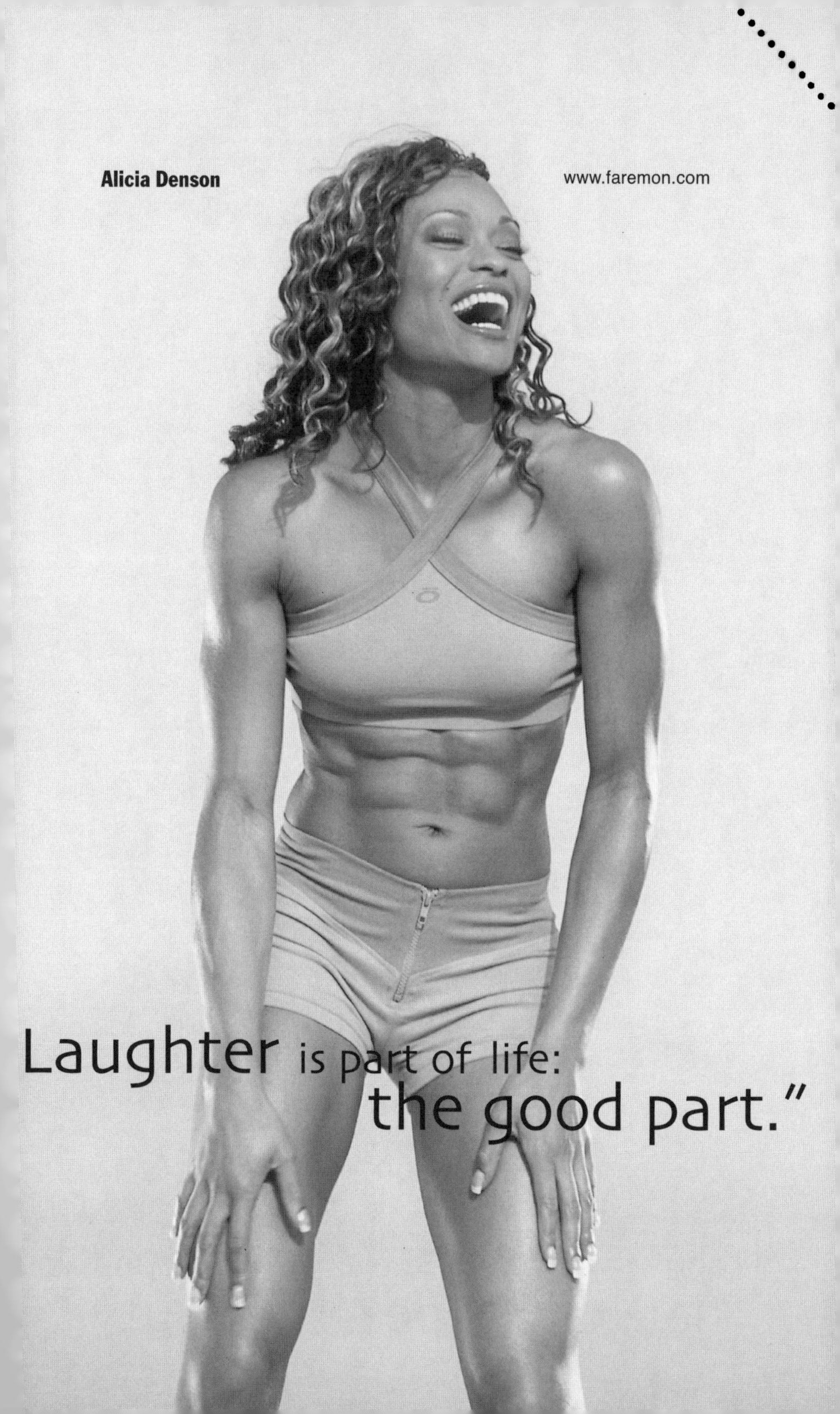

Alicia Denson
www.faremon.com
Laughter is part of life:
the good part."

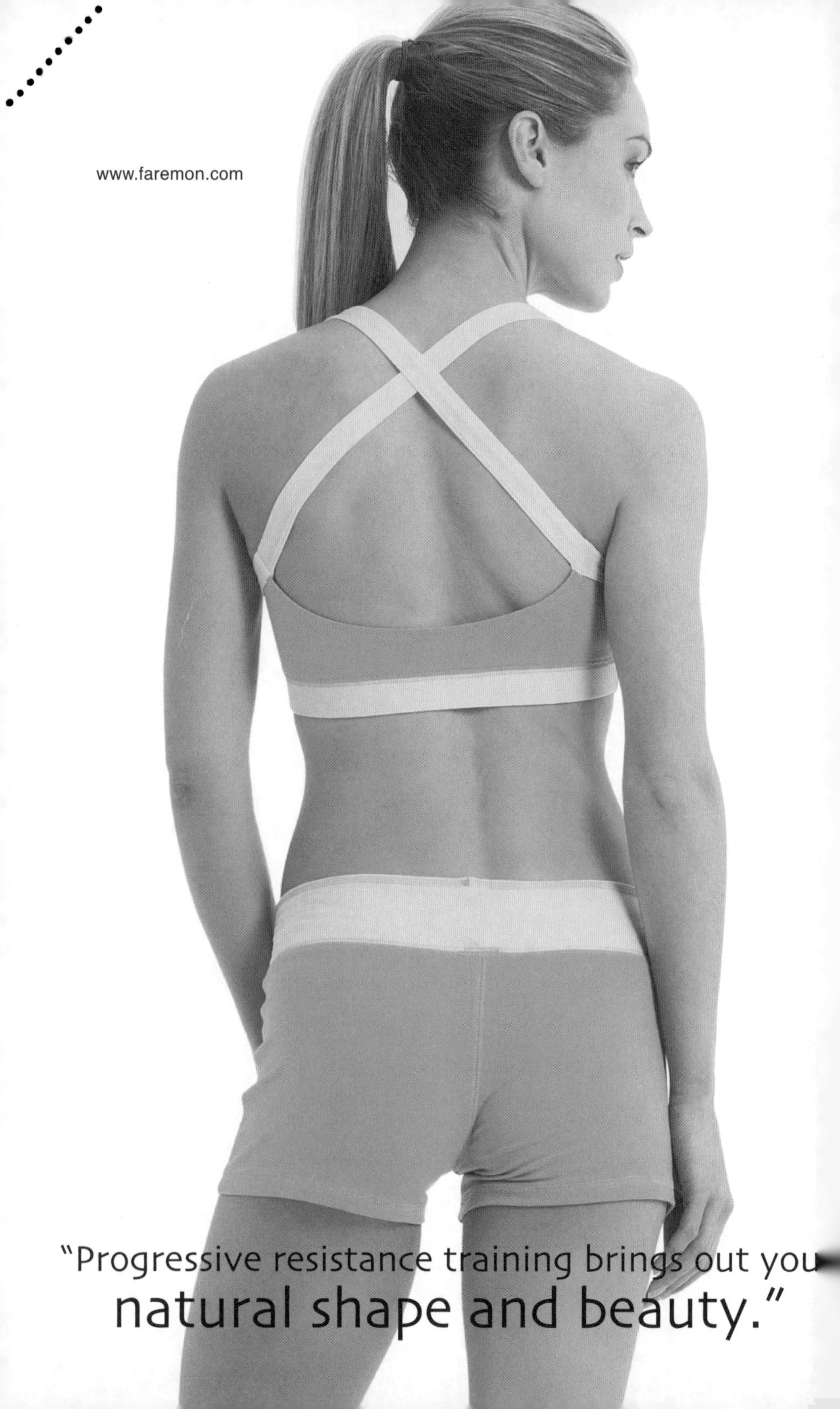
www.faremon.com
“Progressive resistance training brings out you
natural shape and beauty.”

DATE:	SET 1	SET 2	SET 3	SET 4	SET 5	SET 6	SET 7	SET 8
EXERCISE	WEIGHT	WEIGHT	WEIGHT	WEIGHT	WEIGHT	WEIGHT	WEIGHT	WEIGHT
	REPS	REPS	REPS	REPS	REPS	REPS	REPS	REPS

Cardio/Notes:

DATE:	SET 1	SET 2	SET 3	SET 4	SET 5	SET 6	SET 7	SET 8
EXERCISE	WEIGHT REPS	WEIGHT REPS	WEIGHT REPS	WEIGHT REPS	WEIGHT REPS	WEIGHT REPS	WEIGHT REPS	WEIGHT REPS

Cardio/Notes:

DATE:	SET 1	SET 2	SET 3	SET 4	SET 5	SET 6	SET 7	SET 8
EXERCISE	WEIGHT	WEIGHT	WEIGHT	WEIGHT	WEIGHT	WEIGHT	WEIGHT	WEIGHT
	REPS	REPS	REPS	REPS	REPS	REPS	REPS	REPS

Cardio/Notes:

DATE:	SET 1	SET 2	SET 3	SET 4	SET 5	SET 6	SET 7	SET 8
EXERCISE	WEIGHT	WEIGHT	WEIGHT	WEIGHT	WEIGHT	WEIGHT	WEIGHT	WEIGHT
	REPS	REPS	REPS	REPS	REPS	REPS	REPS	REPS

Cardio/Notes:

DATE:	SET 1	SET 2	SET 3	SET 4	SET 5	SET 6	SET 7	SET 8
EXERCISE	WEIGHT	WEIGHT	WEIGHT	WEIGHT	WEIGHT	WEIGHT	WEIGHT	WEIGHT
	REPS	REPS	REPS	REPS	REPS	REPS	REPS	REPS

Cardio/Notes:

DATE:	SET 1	SET 2	SET 3	SET 4	SET 5	SET 6	SET 7	SET 8
EXERCISE	WEIGHT REPS	WEIGHT REPS	WEIGHT REPS	WEIGHT REPS	WEIGHT REPS	WEIGHT REPS	WEIGHT REPS	WEIGHT REPS

Cardio/Notes:

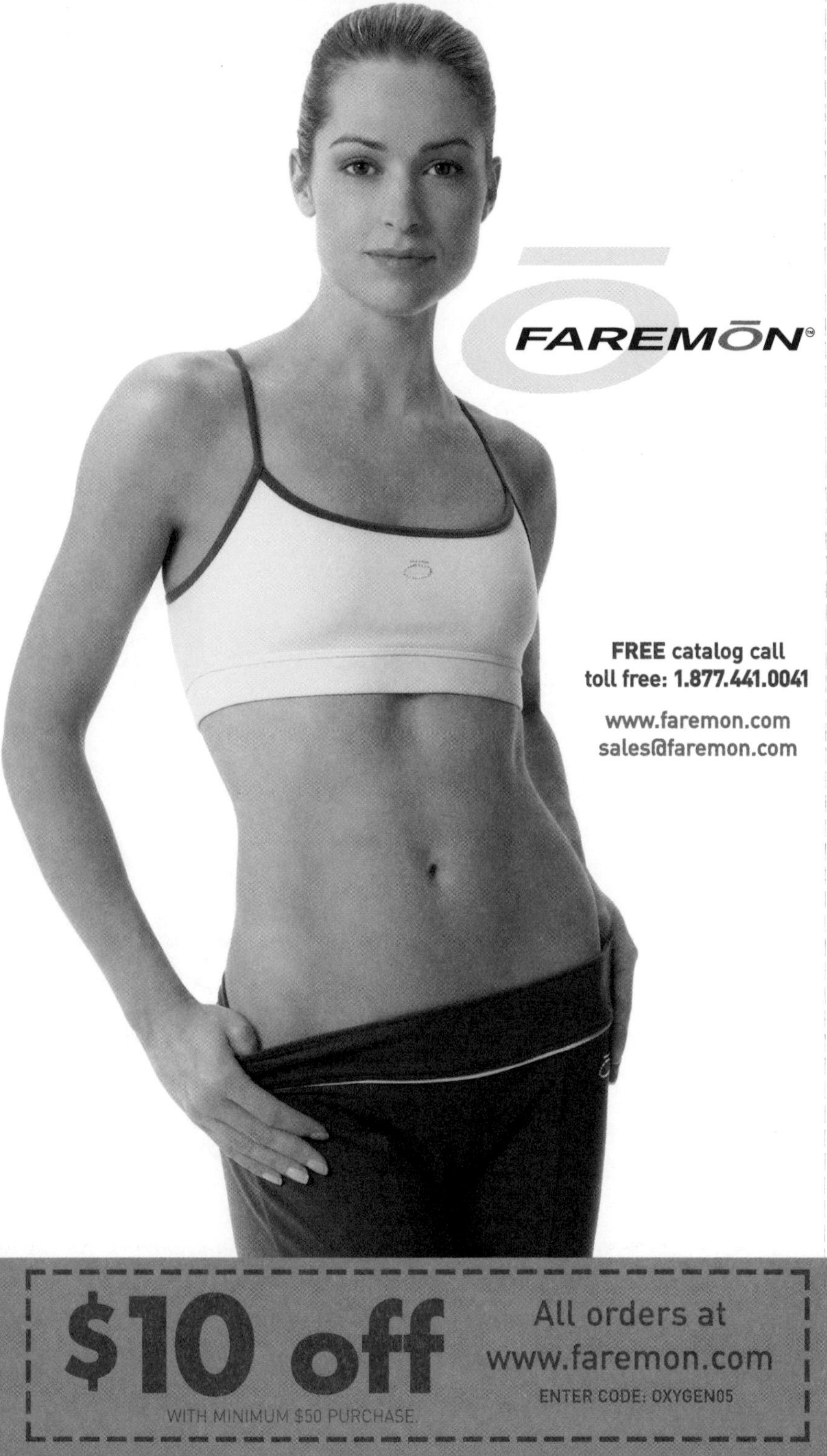
FAREMŌN
FREE catalog call
toll free: 1.877.441.0041
www.faremon.com
sales@faremon.com
$10 off
WITH MINIMUM $50 PURCHASE.
All orders at
www.faremon.com
ENTER CODE: OXYGEN05

DATE:	SET 1	SET 2	SET 3	SET 4	SET 5	SET 6	SET 7	SET 8
EXERCISE	WEIGHT	WEIGHT	WEIGHT	WEIGHT	WEIGHT	WEIGHT	WEIGHT	WEIGHT
	REPS	REPS	REPS	REPS	REPS	REPS	REPS	REPS

Cardio/Notes:

DATE:	SET 1	SET 2	SET 3	SET 4	SET 5	SET 6	SET 7	SET 8
EXERCISE	WEIGHT REPS	WEIGHT REPS	WEIGHT REPS	WEIGHT REPS	WEIGHT REPS	WEIGHT REPS	WEIGHT REPS	WEIGHT REPS

Cardio/Notes:

DATE:	SET 1	SET 2	SET 3	SET 4	SET 5	SET 6	SET 7	SET 8
EXERCISE	WEIGHT REPS	WEIGHT REPS	WEIGHT REPS	WEIGHT REPS	WEIGHT REPS	WEIGHT REPS	WEIGHT REPS	WEIGHT REPS

Cardio/Notes:

DATE:	SET 1	SET 2	SET 3	SET 4	SET 5	SET 6	SET 7	SET 8
EXERCISE	WEIGHT REPS	WEIGHT REPS	WEIGHT REPS	WEIGHT REPS	WEIGHT REPS	WEIGHT REPS	WEIGHT REPS	WEIGHT REPS

Cardio/Notes:

DATE:	SET 1	SET 2	SET 3	SET 4	SET 5	SET 6	SET 7	SET 8
EXERCISE	WEIGHT	WEIGHT	WEIGHT	WEIGHT	WEIGHT	WEIGHT	WEIGHT	WEIGHT
	REPS	REPS	REPS	REPS	REPS	REPS	REPS	REPS

ardio/Notes:

DATE:	SET 1	SET 2	SET 3	SET 4	SET 5	SET 6	SET 7	SET 8
EXERCISE	WEIGHT	WEIGHT	WEIGHT	WEIGHT	WEIGHT	WEIGHT	WEIGHT	WEIGHT
	REPS	REPS	REPS	REPS	REPS	REPS	REPS	REPS

Cardio/Notes:

DATE:	SET 1	SET 2	SET 3	SET 4	SET 5	SET 6	SET 7	SET 8
EXERCISE	WEIGHT	WEIGHT	WEIGHT	WEIGHT	WEIGHT	WEIGHT	WEIGHT	WEIGHT
	REPS	REPS	REPS	REPS	REPS	REPS	REPS	REPS

ardio/Notes:

DATE:	SET 1	SET 2	SET 3	SET 4	SET 5	SET 6	SET 7	SET 8
EXERCISE	WEIGHT / REPS	WEIGHT / REPS	WEIGHT / REPS	WEIGHT / REPS	WEIGHT / REPS	WEIGHT / REPS	WEIGHT / REPS	WEIGH / REPS

Cardio/Notes:

DATE:	SET 1	SET 2	SET 3	SET 4	SET 5	SET 6	SET 7	SET 8
EXERCISE	WEIGHT	WEIGHT	WEIGHT	WEIGHT	WEIGHT	WEIGHT	WEIGHT	WEIGHT
	REPS	REPS	REPS	REPS	REPS	REPS	REPS	REPS

Cardio/Notes:

DATE:	SET 1	SET 2	SET 3	SET 4	SET 5	SET 6	SET 7	SET 8
EXERCISE	WEIGHT REPS	WEIGHT REPS	WEIGHT REPS	WEIGHT REPS	WEIGHT REPS	WEIGHT REPS	WEIGHT REPS	WEIGHT REPS

Cardio/Notes:

DATE:	SET 1	SET 2	SET 3	SET 4	SET 5	SET 6	SET 7	SET 8
EXERCISE	WEIGHT	WEIGHT	WEIGHT	WEIGHT	WEIGHT	WEIGHT	WEIGHT	WEIGHT
	REPS	REPS	REPS	REPS	REPS	REPS	REPS	REPS

ardio/Notes:

DATE:	SET 1	SET 2	SET 3	SET 4	SET 5	SET 6	SET 7	SET 8
EXERCISE	WEIGHT	WEIGHT	WEIGHT	WEIGHT	WEIGHT	WEIGHT	WEIGHT	WEIGH
	REPS	REPS	REPS	REPS	REPS	REPS	REPS	REPS

Cardio/Notes:

DATE:	SET 1	SET 2	SET 3	SET 4	SET 5	SET 6	SET 7	SET 8
EXERCISE	WEIGHT	WEIGHT	WEIGHT	WEIGHT	WEIGHT	WEIGHT	WEIGHT	WEIGHT
	REPS	REPS	REPS	REPS	REPS	REPS	REPS	REPS

Cardio/Notes:

DATE:

EXERCISE	SET 1	SET 2	SET 3	SET 4	SET 5	SET 6	SET 7	SET 8
	WEIGHT / REPS	WEIGHT / REPS	WEIGHT / REPS	WEIGHT / REPS	WEIGHT / REPS	WEIGHT / REPS	WEIGHT / REPS	WEIGHT / REPS

Cardio/Notes:

DATE:	SET 1	SET 2	SET 3	SET 4	SET 5	SET 6	SET 7	SET 8
EXERCISE	WEIGHT REPS	WEIGHT REPS	WEIGHT REPS	WEIGHT REPS	WEIGHT REPS	WEIGHT REPS	WEIGHT REPS	WEIGHT REPS

Cardio/Notes:

DATE:

EXERCISE	SET 1	SET 2	SET 3	SET 4	SET 5	SET 6	SET 7	SET 8
	WEIGHT	WEIGHT	WEIGHT	WEIGHT	WEIGHT	WEIGHT	WEIGHT	WEIGHT
	REPS	REPS	REPS	REPS	REPS	REPS	REPS	REPS

Cardio/Notes:

DATE:	SET 1	SET 2	SET 3	SET 4	SET 5	SET 6	SET 7	SET 8
EXERCISE	WEIGHT REPS	WEIGHT REPS	WEIGHT REPS	WEIGHT REPS	WEIGHT REPS	WEIGHT REPS	WEIGHT REPS	WEIGHT REPS

Cardio/Notes:

DATE:

EXERCISE	SET 1	SET 2	SET 3	SET 4	SET 5	SET 6	SET 7	SET 8
	WEIGHT REPS	WEIGHT REPS	WEIGHT REPS	WEIGHT REPS	WEIGHT REPS	WEIGHT REPS	WEIGHT REPS	WEIGHT REPS

Cardio/Notes:

DATE:	SET 1	SET 2	SET 3	SET 4	SET 5	SET 6	SET 7	SET 8
EXERCISE	WEIGHT	WEIGHT	WEIGHT	WEIGHT	WEIGHT	WEIGHT	WEIGHT	WEIGHT
	REPS	REPS	REPS	REPS	REPS	REPS	REPS	REPS

Cardio/Notes:

DATE:	SET 1	SET 2	SET 3	SET 4	SET 5	SET 6	SET 7	SET 8
EXERCISE	WEIGHT	WEIGHT	WEIGHT	WEIGHT	WEIGHT	WEIGHT	WEIGHT	WEIGHT
	REPS	REPS	REPS	REPS	REPS	REPS	REPS	REPS

Cardio/Notes:

DATE:	SET 1	SET 2	SET 3	SET 4	SET 5	SET 6	SET 7	SET 8
EXERCISE	WEIGHT	WEIGHT	WEIGHT	WEIGHT	WEIGHT	WEIGHT	WEIGHT	WEIGHT
	REPS	REPS	REPS	REPS	REPS	REPS	REPS	REPS

Cardio/Notes:

DATE:

EXERCISE	SET 1	SET 2	SET 3	SET 4	SET 5	SET 6	SET 7	SET 8
	WEIGHT	WEIGHT	WEIGHT	WEIGHT	WEIGHT	WEIGHT	WEIGHT	WEIGHT
	REPS	REPS	REPS	REPS	REPS	REPS	REPS	REPS

Cardio/Notes:

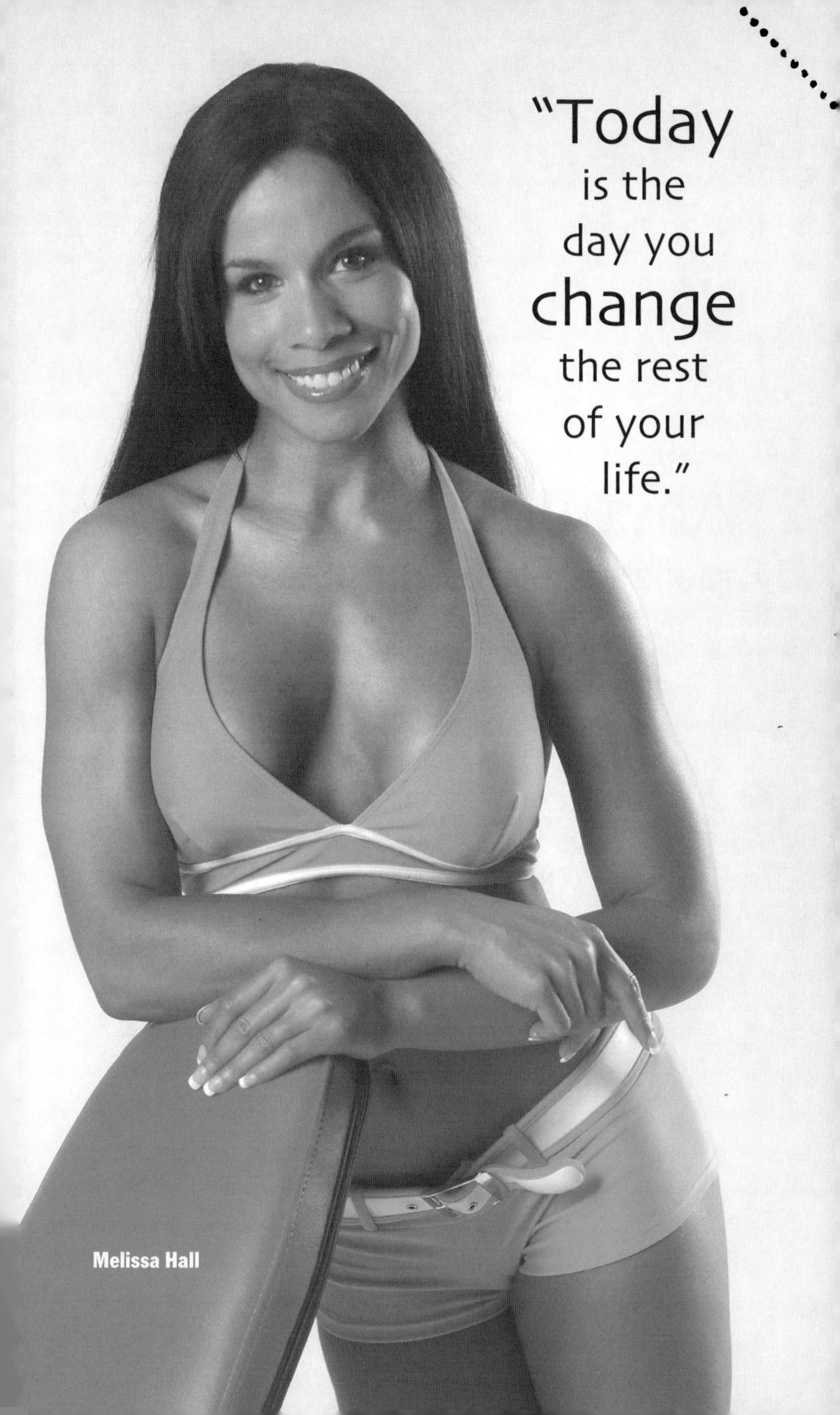
"Today is the day you change the rest of your life."
Melissa Hall

"Anything you can visualize is possible."

Rady Ouzounova

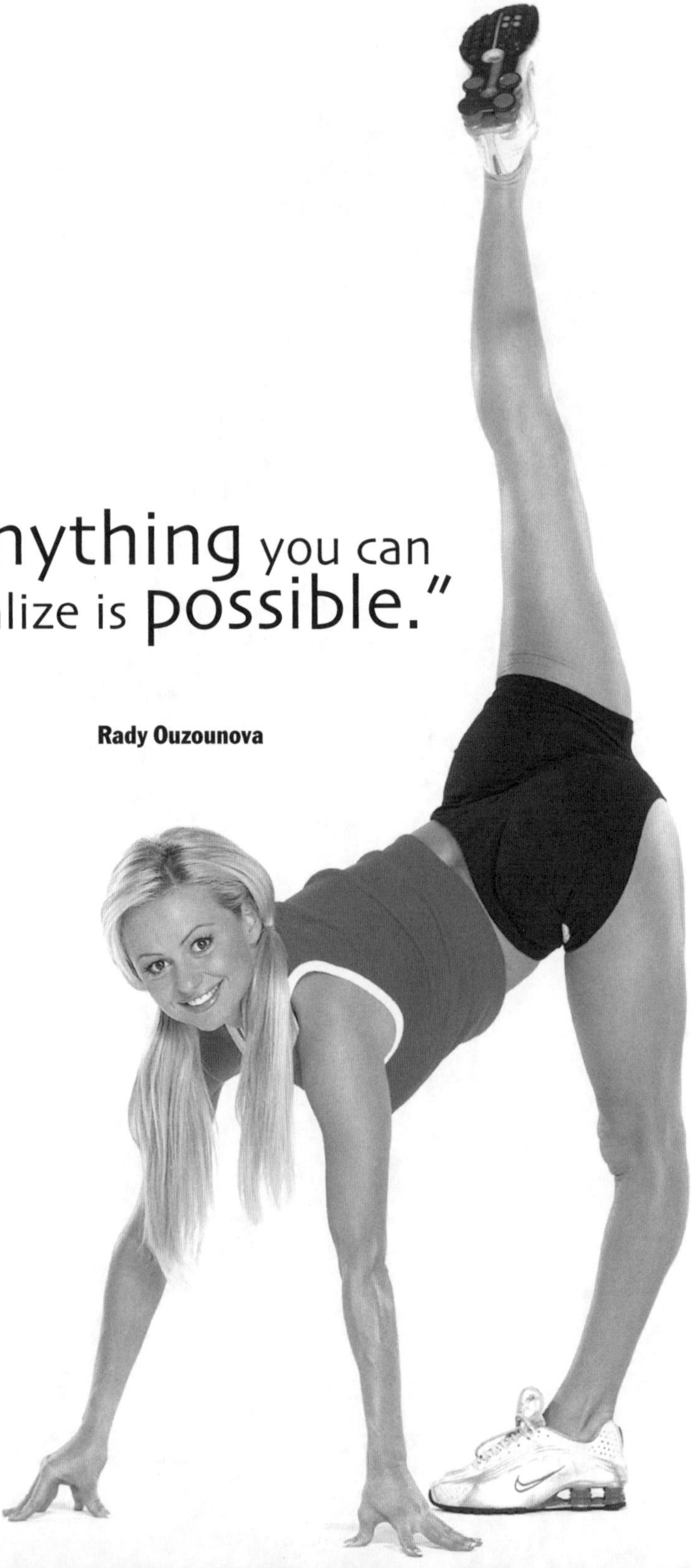

DATE:	SET 1	SET 2	SET 3	SET 4	SET 5	SET 6	SET 7	SET 8
EXERCISE	WEIGHT	WEIGHT	WEIGHT	WEIGHT	WEIGHT	WEIGHT	WEIGHT	WEIGHT
	REPS	REPS	REPS	REPS	REPS	REPS	REPS	REPS

Cardio/Notes:

DATE:	SET 1	SET 2	SET 3	SET 4	SET 5	SET 6	SET 7	SET 8
EXERCISE	WEIGHT	WEIGHT	WEIGHT	WEIGHT	WEIGHT	WEIGHT	WEIGHT	WEIGHT
	REPS	REPS	REPS	REPS	REPS	REPS	REPS	REPS

Cardio/Notes:

DATE:	SET 1	SET 2	SET 3	SET 4	SET 5	SET 6	SET 7	SET 8
EXERCISE	WEIGHT	WEIGHT	WEIGHT	WEIGHT	WEIGHT	WEIGHT	WEIGHT	WEIGHT
	REPS	REPS	REPS	REPS	REPS	REPS	REPS	REPS

Cardio/Notes:

DATE:	SET 1	SET 2	SET 3	SET 4	SET 5	SET 6	SET 7	SET 8
EXERCISE	WEIGHT	WEIGHT	WEIGHT	WEIGHT	WEIGHT	WEIGHT	WEIGHT	WEIGHT
	REPS	REPS	REPS	REPS	REPS	REPS	REPS	REPS

Cardio/Notes:

DATE:	SET 1	SET 2	SET 3	SET 4	SET 5	SET 6	SET 7	SET 8
EXERCISE	WEIGHT REPS	WEIGHT REPS	WEIGHT REPS	WEIGHT REPS	WEIGHT REPS	WEIGHT REPS	WEIGHT REPS	WEIGHT REPS

Cardio/Notes:

DATE:	SET 1	SET 2	SET 3	SET 4	SET 5	SET 6	SET 7	SET 8
EXERCISE	WEIGHT REPS	WEIGHT REPS	WEIGHT REPS	WEIGHT REPS	WEIGHT REPS	WEIGHT REPS	WEIGHT REPS	WEIGHT REPS

Cardio/Notes:

DATE:	SET 1	SET 2	SET 3	SET 4	SET 5	SET 6	SET 7	SET 8
EXERCISE	WEIGHT	WEIGHT	WEIGHT	WEIGHT	WEIGHT	WEIGHT	WEIGHT	WEIGHT
	REPS	REPS	REPS	REPS	REPS	REPS	REPS	REPS

Cardio/Notes:

DATE:	SET 1	SET 2	SET 3	SET 4	SET 5	SET 6	SET 7	SET 8
EXERCISE	WEIGHT	WEIGHT	WEIGHT	WEIGHT	WEIGHT	WEIGHT	WEIGHT	WEIGHT
	REPS	REPS	REPS	REPS	REPS	REPS	REPS	REPS

Cardio/Notes:

DATE:	SET 1	SET 2	SET 3	SET 4	SET 5	SET 6	SET 7	SET 8
EXERCISE	WEIGHT	WEIGHT	WEIGHT	WEIGHT	WEIGHT	WEIGHT	WEIGHT	WEIGHT
	REPS	REPS	REPS	REPS	REPS	REPS	REPS	REPS

Cardio/Notes:

DATE:	SET 1	SET 2	SET 3	SET 4	SET 5	SET 6	SET 7	SET 8
EXERCISE	WEIGHT	WEIGHT	WEIGHT	WEIGHT	WEIGHT	WEIGHT	WEIGHT	WEIGHT
	REPS	REPS	REPS	REPS	REPS	REPS	REPS	REPS

Cardio/Notes:

DATE:	SET 1	SET 2	SET 3	SET 4	SET 5	SET 6	SET 7	SET 8
EXERCISE	WEIGHT	WEIGHT	WEIGHT	WEIGHT	WEIGHT	WEIGHT	WEIGHT	WEIGHT
	REPS	REPS	REPS	REPS	REPS	REPS	REPS	REPS

Cardio/Notes:

DATE:	SET 1	SET 2	SET 3	SET 4	SET 5	SET 6	SET 7	SET 8
EXERCISE	WEIGHT	WEIGHT	WEIGHT	WEIGHT	WEIGHT	WEIGHT	WEIGHT	WEIGHT
	REPS	REPS	REPS	REPS	REPS	REPS	REPS	REPS

Cardio/Notes:

DATE:	SET 1	SET 2	SET 3	SET 4	SET 5	SET 6	SET 7	SET 8
EXERCISE	WEIGHT REPS	WEIGHT REPS	WEIGHT REPS	WEIGHT REPS	WEIGHT REPS	WEIGHT REPS	WEIGHT REPS	WEIGHT REPS

Cardio/Notes:

DATE:

EXERCISE	SET 1	SET 2	SET 3	SET 4	SET 5	SET 6	SET 7	SET 8
	WEIGHT	WEIGHT	WEIGHT	WEIGHT	WEIGHT	WEIGHT	WEIGHT	WEIGHT
	REPS	REPS	REPS	REPS	REPS	REPS	REPS	REPS

Cardio/Notes:

DATE:	SET 1	SET 2	SET 3	SET 4	SET 5	SET 6	SET 7	SET 8
EXERCISE	WEIGHT	WEIGHT	WEIGHT	WEIGHT	WEIGHT	WEIGHT	WEIGHT	WEIGHT
	REPS	REPS	REPS	REPS	REPS	REPS	REPS	REPS

Cardio/Notes:

DATE: EXERCISE	SET 1	SET 2	SET 3	SET 4	SET 5	SET 6	SET 7	SET 8
	WEIGHT	WEIGHT	WEIGHT	WEIGHT	WEIGHT	WEIGHT	WEIGHT	WEIGHT
	REPS	REPS	REPS	REPS	REPS	REPS	REPS	REPS

Cardio/Notes:

DATE:	SET 1	SET 2	SET 3	SET 4	SET 5	SET 6	SET 7	SET 8
EXERCISE	WEIGHT REPS	WEIGHT REPS	WEIGHT REPS	WEIGHT REPS	WEIGHT REPS	WEIGHT REPS	WEIGHT REPS	WEIGHT REPS

Cardio/Notes:

DATE:	SET 1	SET 2	SET 3	SET 4	SET 5	SET 6	SET 7	SET 8
EXERCISE	WEIGHT REPS	WEIGHT REPS	WEIGHT REPS	WEIGHT REPS	WEIGHT REPS	WEIGHT REPS	WEIGHT REPS	WEIGHT REPS

Cardio/Notes:

DATE:	SET 1	SET 2	SET 3	SET 4	SET 5	SET 6	SET 7	SET 8
EXERCISE	WEIGHT REPS	WEIGHT REPS	WEIGHT REPS	WEIGHT REPS	WEIGHT REPS	WEIGHT REPS	WEIGHT REPS	WEIGHT REPS

Cardio/Notes:

DATE:

EXERCISE	SET 1	SET 2	SET 3	SET 4	SET 5	SET 6	SET 7	SET 8
	WEIGHT	WEIGHT	WEIGHT	WEIGHT	WEIGHT	WEIGHT	WEIGHT	WEIGHT
	REPS	REPS	REPS	REPS	REPS	REPS	REPS	REPS

Cardio/Notes:

DATE:	SET 1	SET 2	SET 3	SET 4	SET 5	SET 6	SET 7	SET 8
EXERCISE	WEIGHT REPS	WEIGHT REPS	WEIGHT REPS	WEIGHT REPS	WEIGHT REPS	WEIGHT REPS	WEIGHT REPS	WEIGHT REPS

Cardio/Notes:

DATE:

EXERCISE	SET 1	SET 2	SET 3	SET 4	SET 5	SET 6	SET 7	SET 8
	WEIGHT REPS	WEIGHT REPS	WEIGHT REPS	WEIGHT REPS	WEIGHT REPS	WEIGHT REPS	WEIGHT REPS	WEIGHT REPS

Cardio/Notes:

"Determination to succeed is key."

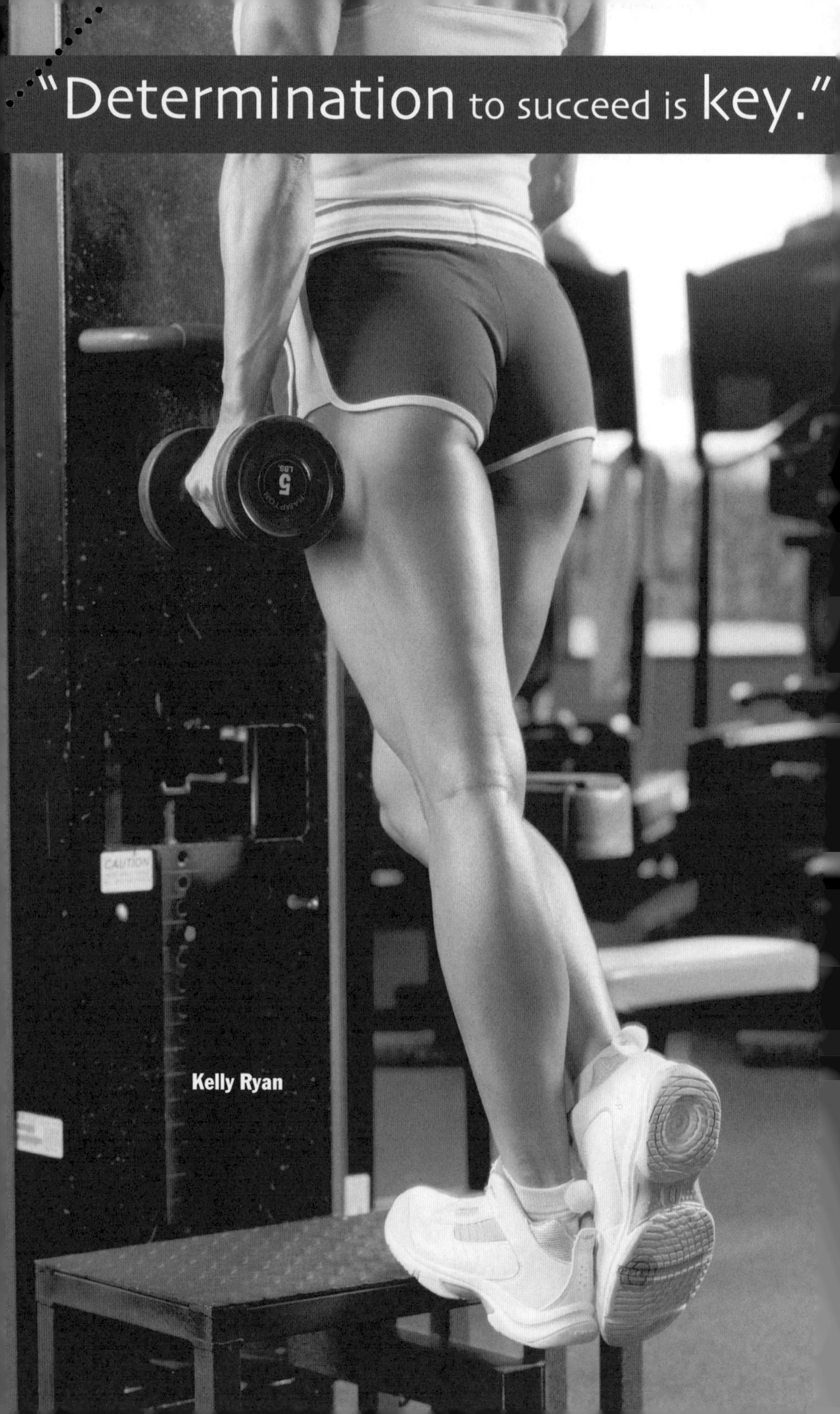

Kelly Ryan

Calculating Intensity Levels

Monitor the intensity of your cardio workouts by checking your heart rate regularly. The least expensive method is to feel the pulse in an artery on your wrist or throat. Count the number of heart beats for 10 seconds, then multiply the 10-second value by 6. This allows for a more accurate reading as your pulse drops significantly within one minute of exercise cooldown.

Everyone responds to exercise differently; however, the following heart-rate ranges can act as a guide during your cardio workouts.

Beginners: aim for 55-65% of MHR
Intermediates: aim for 65-75% of MHR
Advanced: aim for 75-85% of MHR

FORMULA FOR HEART-RATE VALUES:

MEN: 220 - your age = MHR (maximum heart rate)
WOMEN: 226 - your age = MHR

Multiply your maximum heart rate (MHR) by your desired intensity level (% of MHR) to find the optimal number of heart beats per minute.

HEART-RATE TABLE

			% of MHR							
AGE	**MHR**		**55%**		**65%**		**75%**		**85%**	
20	*206*	200	*113*	112	*134*	130	*155*	150	*175*	170
25	*201*	195	*111*	107	*131*	127	*151*	146	*171*	166
30	*196*	190	*108*	105	*127*	123	*147*	143	*167*	162
35	*191*	185	*105*	102	*124*	120	*143*	139	*162*	157
40	*186*	180	*102*	99	*121*	117	*140*	135	*158*	153
45	*181*	175	*100*	96	*118*	114	*136*	131	*154*	149
50	*176*	170	*97*	94	*114*	110	*132*	128	*150*	145
55	*171*	165	*94*	91	*111*	107	*128*	124	*145*	140
60	*166*	160	*91*	88	*108*	104	*125*	120	*141*	136
65	*161*	155	*89*	85	*105*	101	*121*	116	*137*	132
70	*156*	150	*86*	83	*101*	97	*117*	113	*133*	128

** Grey areas represent women's values.*

Muscle Groups

Anterior View

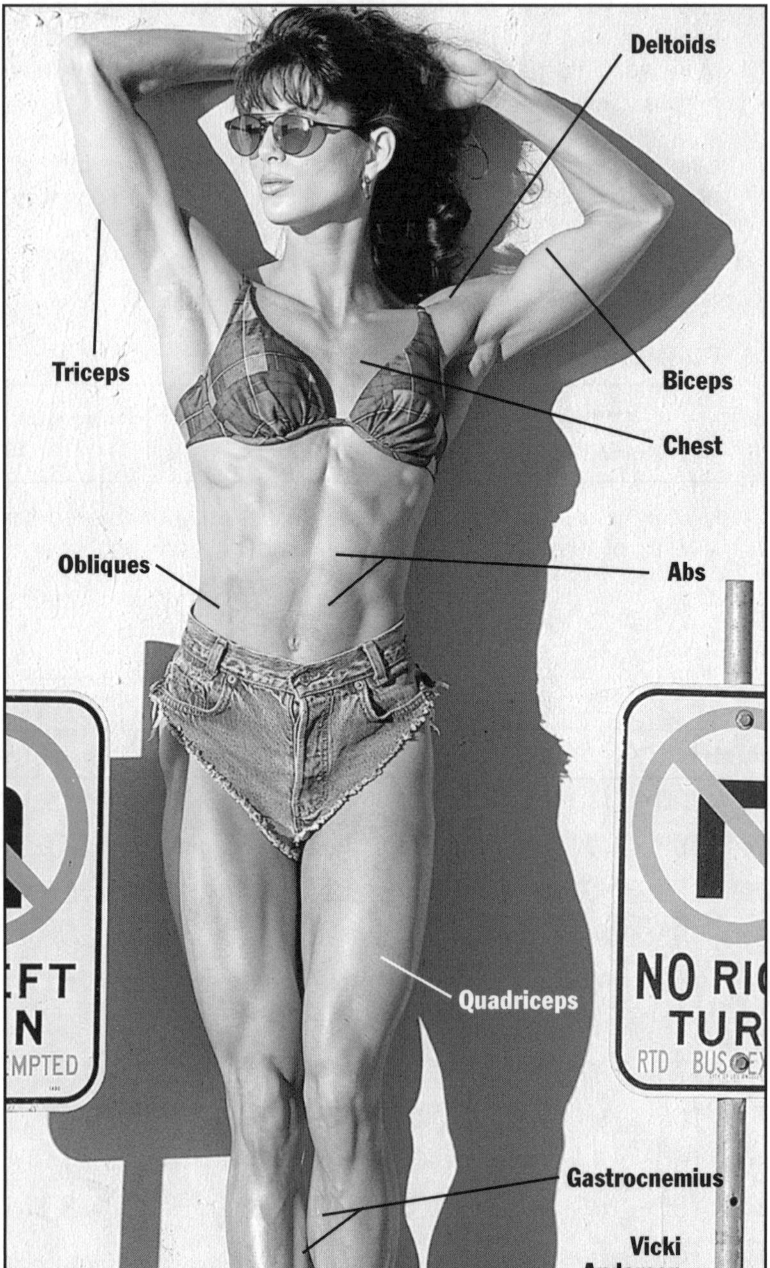

Posterior View

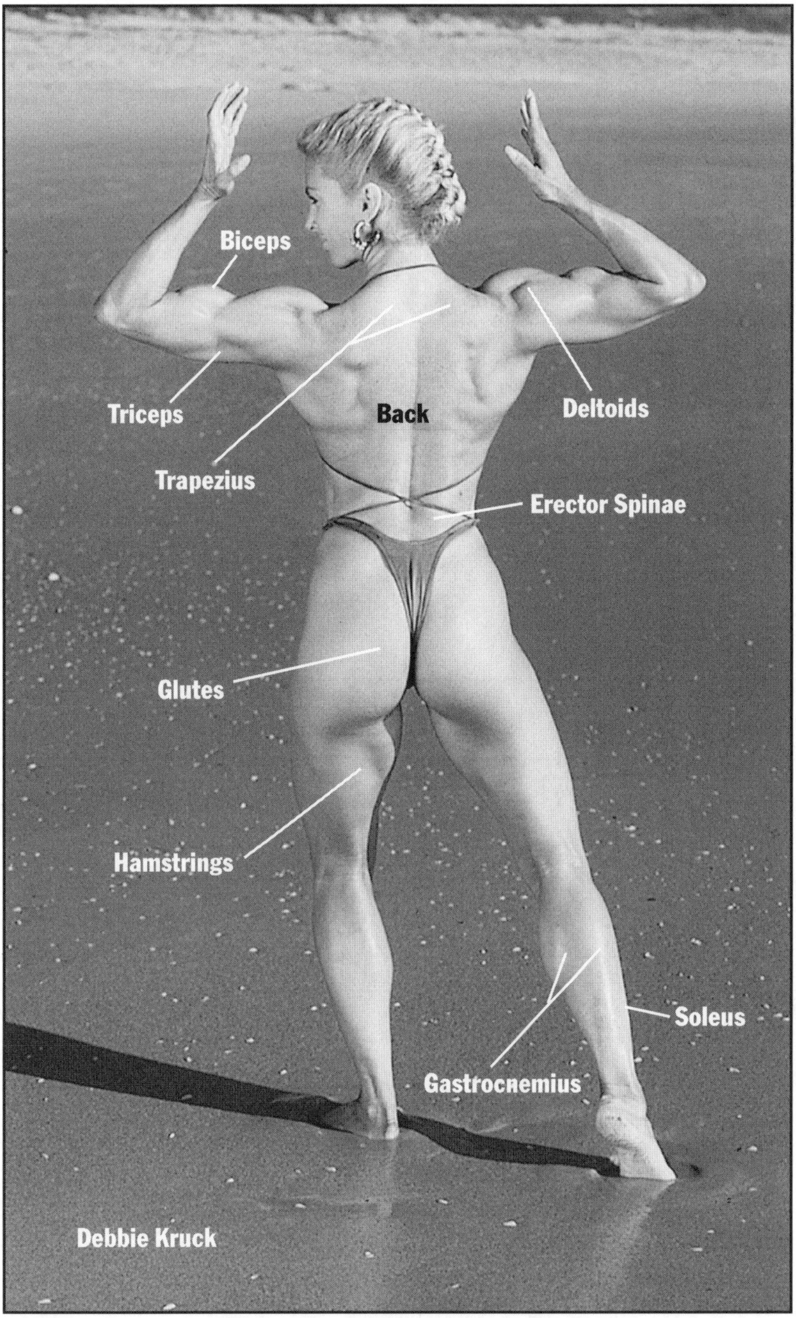

Personal Data

	DATE: ___________	DATE: ___________	DATE: ___________
Weight:			
Bodyfat %:			
MEASUREMENTS			
Chest:			
Waist:			
Hips:			
Thigh:			
Right Arm – relaxed:			
– flexed:			
Left Arm – relaxed:			
– flexed:			
Right Calf:			
Left Calf:			
Neck:			
Forearm:			

Record measurements approximately every 30 days.

Personal Data

	DATE: ________	DATE: ________	DATE: ________
Weight:			
Bodyfat %:			
MEASUREMENTS			
Chest:			
Waist:			
Hips:			
Thigh:			
Right Arm – relaxed:			
– flexed:			
Left Arm – relaxed:			
– flexed:			
Right Calf:			
Left Calf:			
Neck:			
Forearm:			

Record measurements approximately every 30 days.

Goals and Reminders

January

February

March

April

May

June

Goals and Reminders

July

August

September

October

November

December

Metric Conversions

Symbol	When You Know	Multiply By	To Find	Symbol
LENGTH				
in	inches	2.54	centimeters	cm
ft	feet	30	centimeters	cm
yd	yards	0.9	meters	m
mi	miles	1.6	kilometers	km
mm	millimeters	0.04	inches	in
cm	centimeters	0.4	inches	in
m	meters	3.3	feet	ft
m	meters	1.1	yards	yd
km	kilometers	0.6	miles	mi
WEIGHT				
oz	ounces	28	grams	g
lb	pounds	0.45	kilograms	kg
g	grams	0.035	ounce	oz
kg	kilograms	2.2	pounds	lb
VOLUME				
tsp	teaspoons	5	milliliters	ml
tbsp	tablespoons	15	milliliters	ml
fl oz	fluid ounces	30	milliliters	ml
c	cups	0.24	liters	l
pt	pints	0.47	liters	l
qt	quarts	0.95	liters	l
ml	milliliters	0.03	fluid ounces	fl oz
l	liters	2.1	pints	pt
l	liters	1.06	quarts	qt

TEMPERATURE

°C = (°F – 32) x .555

°F = (°C x 1.8) + 32

Phone Numbers

Name and Address	Telephone

Notes